EIGHTYSOMETHINGS

A Practical Guide to Letting Go, Aging Well, and Finding Unexpected Happiness

KATHARINE ESTY, PhD

Skyhorse Publishing

Skyhorse Publishing books may be purchased in bulk at special discounts for sales promotion,
corporate gifts, fund-raising, or educational purposes. Special editions can also be created to
specifications. For details, contact the Special Sales Department, Skyhorse Publishing,
307 West 36th Street, 11th Floor, New York, NY 10018 or info@skyhorsepublishing.com.

Skyhorse® and Skyhorse Publishing® are registered trademarks of Skyhorse Publishing, Inc.®,
a Delaware corporation.

Visit our website at www.skyhorsepublishing.com.

10 9 8 7 6 5 4 3 2 1

Library of Congress Cataloging-in-Publication Data is available on file.

Cover design by Paul Qualcom

Print ISBN: 978-1-5107-7120-8
Ebook ISBN: 978-1-5107-4319-9

Printed in the United States of America

CONTENTS

INTRODUCTION

Each ten years of a life has its own fortune, its own hopes, its own desires.

—Goethe

For many people in their seventies, life rolls along as it always has. They continue to play tennis and golf and trek in the Himalayas. They spend time at the gym and go south in the winter. They work at jobs and provide care to grandchildren. At my husband John's seventy-fifth birthday party, he told family and friends, "I feel like a young man who has a few little things wrong with him." At that point, he had arthritis, a sore hip, and some early signs of kidney problems. I, unlike him at seventy-five, had no real health issues at all and all the energy that I needed to keep doing what I wanted.

But at eighty, I began to feel quite different. I felt I had entered a strange and foreign country without a map or a guide. I had a moment while attempting to climb a mountain that made me realize I was old. Several of my good friends had died and this was not only sad for me but scary. I began to worry about my own health and even my mortality. Could I maintain my busy, well, frantic lifestyle? Was I doing too much and putting myself at risk? I wondered what life was really like for others in their eighties. Were there predictable patterns, shifts and transitions? Or did everyone age in their own unique way?

To learn more about being eighty, I read a number of books about aging and adult development over the lifespan. I soon discovered it was not easy to tease out information just about people in their eighties. People sixty-five to a hundred are usually lumped together. I realized that if I wanted to learn more about what it is like to be an eightysomething, I would have to do some research of my own.

I began by looking at my own family. Neither of my parents made it past age seventy-one. The same for my grandfathers. Not much help there. But what about my grandmothers?

My maternal grandmother, who died at ninety-three, fell and broke her hip when she was eighty-one and she never walked after that. Although she remained cheerful, being old and bedridden looked like an awful way to live.

My paternal grandmother, who lived to eighty-eight, had a happier story. She seemed to be enjoying her life and her garden to the end. However, I found her long conversations about her digestive system, gene-alogy, and family members I had never known to be incredibly boring. I knew she loved me, but she was a bit harsh about writing thank-you notes and table manners. I thought as a child, if that is what being in your eighties is like, well, I just do not want to grow old.

I still felt that way years later when I myself was eighty and embarking on this project. Is that all there is to life when you are old? From my research, I soon learned that being in the eighties today is different from the past. First, because there are suddenly many more eightysomethings than ever before, almost ten million in the United States alone. And sec-ond, due to modern medicine, many of them are living in relatively good health and without pain. This opened up possibilities for eightysome-things' lives that had not yet been explored. I wanted to find out about them.

I decided to interview people in their eighties living in all kinds of cir-cumstances. Over the next three years I spoke with 128 eightysomethings as well as twenty-six adult children of eightysomethings. The people in their eighties that I spoke with were diverse by gender, class, race, ethnicity, level of disability, economic level, and sexual orientation. They lived alone, with spouses, and with children, in their own homes, in retirement communities, and in nursing homes. About half of my interviews were in person and the other half by phone—enabling me to talk with people in every region of the country. I traveled to California, Louisiana, Maine, Rhode Island, Virginia, Ohio, New York, and Connecticut. I was deeply touched by the process of conducting these interviews as people told me about their lives and their inner worlds. And I was changed myself.

Besides my interviews, I had other sources of information for the book. I brought my thirty years of experience as a psychotherapist in private practice. I also relied on my experience in business—coaching managers and executives on personal effectiveness and facilitating strategic planning. Then I drew on my observations of all I have seen and heard at my retirement community over the last eight years. There were also my experiences with shifting relationships within my family as I aged. And, finally, I used my observations of my own aging these last four years as an eightysomething.

I learned that, yes, there are important transitions that eightysomethings experience. Although predictable, they still often come as a surprise and are unsettling. There are many kinds of losses, expected and unexpected, that must be grieved, but there are also new possibilities that emerge. But most surprising of all, most of the eightysomethings whom I interviewed reported that they were happy, some of them happier than they have ever been in their entire lives. From those I spoke with, I came to understand how this could possibly be true. *Eightysomethings* is a practical guide to the unfamiliar landscape of old age that illuminates pathways for aging well.

READING *EIGHTYSOMETHINGS*

Reading the book provides families of eightysomethings—their children, their grandchildren, their nieces and nephews—with insights they need to understand the eightysomething experience and guidance that can help them relate well to their aging relative. It shines a light on the inner world of people in their eighties and reveals aspects of their lives they rarely talk about. It will help younger readers see what is possible in old age and dispel some of their fears of aging.

For those family members who are in regular contact with an eightysomething, reading the book together, either a chapter or part of a chapter at a time, works well. The book is by topic, so some chapters will be more of a priority to you than others. At the end of each chapter are questions that family member can use as conversation starters. There are also tips for the family that can be discussed with the eightysomething to test the waters to see which ones should be pursued. This book is a thought-provoking read for small groups at churches and all sorts of book groups.

This book provides eightysomethings themselves with the chance to reflect on their experience and learn from the experiences of many others. It is useful at retirement communities and at Councils on Aging. It challenges the negative stereotypes of the elderly that are still accepted by many people despite evidence to the contrary.

NOTE TO READERS

To protect their privacy, I have changed the names of all of those whom I interviewed as well as altering a few of the biographical details in some of the vignettes. Quotes from the interviews have been edited for ease of comprehension.

CHAPTER I

I AM NOT OLD!

It was a Cat Mountain day! We all agreed we should climb the mountain. I was vacationing in the Adirondacks with three of my sons and their families. After a day of rain, the sun was shining—the view would be spectacular. Though I had climbed Cat Mountain many times in my life, I was still glad to hear that the last half-mile of the trail, the very steep path up the mountain, had been improved over the winter.

I started out brimming with good spirits. The path was a bit slippery after the rain and in the first ten minutes I stumbled on a root and scraped my knee on a sharp rock. Nothing serious, just a little bleeding. But I did feel a bit shaky jumping across a narrow brook; my legs didn't work quite right. I pushed on, although I became aware it was getting harder to keep up with the group. *But I am the amazing Gran who still does push-ups. This cannot be a real problem, can it?* An hour later, by the time we reached the last half-mile, the starting point of the steep trail, I found myself out of breath and apprehensive. The path had not been improved. I watched the grandchildren scamper up ahead of me.

As I looked up at that forbidding mountainside, I realized I did not have the energy to attempt going further. I sat down on a stump. My son Dan sat with me as I came to terms with the idea that I was not going to make it to the top. I was crushed. I usually just powered through difficult challenges.

An hour later, waiting for all the others to come down from the mountaintop, I still sat frozen on that stump. But I had begun to put myself

1

back together. *It makes sense that I can't do what I did last year. After all, I'm eighty. Do I think I'm superwoman?* Now here, at last, I was finally coming to terms with reality. I, like everyone else in my generation, was aging. Obviously, I could not go on forever. But clearly, at some level, I had assumed exactly that, that I would go on forever. I was basically okay, I knew, and I was even able to laugh as we discussed my "failure to summit." Yet I knew I would remember that moment, that uncomfortable stump, for the rest of my life as the point in time when I came face to face with my own aging.

Before this event, I had almost always avoided thinking about it. Since neither of my parents had made it to eighty, I felt lucky. But without many role models to guide me into this new territory, I was uncertain what being eighty might mean for me. I just hoped that nothing would change.

As my resistance to thinking about aging lessened, I found myself curious about being eighty. Questions kept floating into my mind. What was it really like for others to be in their eighties? What were the possibilities? What are the facts about eightysomethings? What is known? Soon I was pursuing answers to these and other questions and the quest eventually became this book.

I unearthed some interesting statistics. One out of three people born today in the United States will live to be one hundred. Life expectancy in the United States is seventy-nine years on average.[1] For women it is eighty-one and for men it is seventy-six. When people reach eighty today, their life expectancy at that point is 9.6 more years for women and 8.1 years for men.[2] But the United States has by no means the highest life expectancy in the world. It ranks twenty-sixth among thirty-five industrialized countries. Life expectancy in Japan is eighty-four, with Spain, Italy, and Switzerland not far behind.[3]

There are almost ten million people in their eighties in the United States today. The real story here, though, is that the number of people over eighty is skyrocketing. The over-eighty population is growing significantly faster than the populations of people in their sixties or in their seventies. By 2050, the over-eighty population will have grown to more than thirty million.[4]

Having been so afraid to grow old myself, in denial about my own aging, I now began to wonder just why it is that aging is so dreaded by almost everybody. One answer is obvious: American culture values youth—looking young and acting young. But there are many cultures around the world, such as the Chinese and the Japanese, where old people are revered. Then again, they have been treated badly, too. There have been allegations, mostly in the distant past, of some cultures, such as the Chukchi of Siberia, where old people would be expected to request to be put to death when they were no longer healthy.[5]

Back to the United States today, millions of people spend thousands of hours and thousands of dollars frantically striving to hide the fact that they are aging. Over sixteen billion dollars were spent on facelifts and other cosmetic surgeries in 2016 in the United States.[6] Few of us can avoid the pressure to look young. While I like to think of myself as impervious to advertisements and hype, I have been dyeing my hair for forty years. And, recently, I have found myself avoiding having my picture taken because I feared I would look too old.

So it seems that most of us have negative stereotypes about old people. While stereotypes of a people or group can in theory be both positive and negative, in my research, I came across few positive stereotypes about old people. Here are eight of the commonly held negative beliefs about older people according to an article that appeared in the *Senior Citizen Times*.[7]

Old people are unproductive.
Old people cannot learn.
Older people have no interest in or capacity for sexual activity.
Old people are boring and forgetful.

Old people are grouchy and cantankerous.

Old people are set in their ways and can't change.

Old people are usually sick, weak, and helpless.

Most older people live in institutions.

According to social psychologist Ruth Lamont, stereotypes, though not always true, still have serious consequences. In her analysis of thirty-seven studies about the impact of stereotypes of old people on old people, she found that the performance of older people performing a range of tasks gets worse when they are reminded of these stereotypes. She writes, "We all spend a life-time internalizing stereotypes of ageing until we reach old age ourselves and realize we are the targets of these stereotypes."[8]

The good news is that people who resist these kinds of negative stereotypes and have a positive perception of aging live 7.5 years longer than those with less positive views of aging, according to a study in the *Journal of Personality and Social Psychology*.[9] That finding is stunning. It began to convince me that our attitudes and beliefs about aging shape our experience to a significant degree, much more than most of us can imagine. Attitude may be just as important as our actual health status in terms of our longevity.

To learn what life is really like for people in their eighties, I realized I needed to meet with many eightysomethings and listen to what they had to say. Agatha and Steven were among the first people I interviewed. While they both radiated optimism and reported a positive experience of aging, their lifestyles and circumstances were completely different. I began to see how complicated it was going to be to capture the experience of being eightysomething.

Most days, Agatha, eighty-nine, toots around the countryside near her Providence, Rhode Island retirement community in her sedan. A former nun, Agatha is a tall, regal woman with salt and pepper gray hair and chiseled features—kind of a Katharine Hepburn look-alike. Although she never knew any of her grandparents, her mother instilled in her a great love and respect for older people. By the time Agatha was nine, almost every day her mother would send her around to elderly neighbors in her neighborhood to see if they needed any help. She remembers walking the mile to the grocery store with her elderly neighbor and helping her carry the packages home.

She told me, "I never think about being old and aging. You can moan and groan forever but that's not me. I am starting to slip a little this year, but I still know which side is up. It is harder for me to get in and out of my car, but I am a very good driver." I inquired if she has had any fender benders, thinking about my own somewhat battered car. She said "not a one."

After making the decision to become a nun, Agatha was assigned the job of teacher. Each year or so she was transferred to a new city and given jobs with more and more administrative responsibilities. In her late fifties, when she felt the church had abandoned some of its core principles, she left the sisterhood after thirty years. She began a new life totally on her own. Two years later, she got married, a most unexpected turn of events. When she and her husband moved to a retirement community, she told her husband, "I am not going to volunteer for anything or be in charge of anything ever again." Now a widow, she has stuck to her decision and loves her freedom.

Agatha continued, "It is my nature to be active—I go out every day. Usually I get coffee, see friends, or go to the library." She goes to mass most days and watches it on TV on the days when she doesn't go to church. She sees friends for dinner sometimes and keeps up with her husband's children. "I support what's good, try to be pleasant and helpful. I try to extend myself to the staff and the aides here at the retirement community. I also try and reach out to some of the residents who are cantankerous. But I never make commitments that I can't keep. I am free. I am happy."

What struck me about Agatha was how after a lifetime of duty and service to others she is so clear now about avoiding responsibilities. She revels in the fact there is no one telling her what to do and she is free to do what she wants. This is one of the upsides of being old that rarely gets talked about—that if eightysomethings are still in good health, they may be freer than they have ever been in their lives. Children are usually long since out of the nest and even grandchildren are often no longer young.

Like Agatha, Steven has a positive attitude toward aging despite the fact that he has a type of cancer called chronic myeloid leukemia. At eighty-one, he is painfully thin. His lanky body has shrunk and he is unable to stand up straight. His skin is blueish-white. Before he retired, he ran a business in New Hampshire and coached hockey.

"Growing up," he said in a husky voice, "I revered old people as a source of wisdom. My family emphasized our heritage and told me lots of stories about my grandparents and great-grandparents. One great-grandfather was an abolitionist and another believed in spirits and talked with his dead relatives. My dad was my hero all my life. I always asked for his advice even when I was grown." Now living in his father's house, he tells me, "After he died, I spent several years going through all his papers and files figuring out what to save."

He continued:

I never thought I would make it past sixty because of all the cancer in my family. I was rescued by modern medicine. Actually, I have discovered I am not a retirement person. Going to Florida and playing shuffleboard is not my idea of the good life. I just took a part-time job with a hockey coach at a local college helping him develop his program and recruit some kids for his team. I think this job will keep me alive.

My wife has cancer, too, and my first priority is to stay alive to take care of her. And my second priority is to watch the grandchildren grow and emerge. I have been having so much fun tying trout flies with two grandsons. Last week I had the incredible experience of seeing a bald eagle. I will stay here in my home. They will have to use a block and tackle to get me out.

I was moved by my time with Steven and his courage in the face of his own illness and that of his wife. I saw that, far from making him depressed and despairing, his dire circumstances seemed to be strengthening his spirit. He told me he sees every day as a gift, an extra bonus. So many in his family were not so fortunate.

Not everyone in their eighties is as positive as Steven and Agatha and I need to give the negative and unhappy people their voice, too. Maxine, eighty-five, who is a short, roly-poly woman living in eastern Connecticut, is one of these people. Shaking her head and wiping her long black bangs off her face, she told me:

I never wanted to be eighty. I hate my legs, my legs are fat and my boobs are dragging. Everything is sagging. I have a hernia but I decided not to operate. It doesn't bother me. In my seventies I could do everything I wanted. In my eighties, I have balance problems and I can't do much.

It's time to go. I don't have much money. I have term life and it is running out in four years. I don't care if I have two or three more good years. I should be getting rid of some stuff and I should cancel my expensive cable, but I don't do it. But one good thing, I no longer try to lose weight. I say, "to hell with it."

What struck me most about Maxine is her "to hell with it" attitude. She has given up on taking care of herself and on planning for her last years. And, in that respect she is not that unusual. Most people do not anticipate their aging or plan for the changes they may experience as they age. According to a survey by Bankrate.com, 65 percent of Americans save little or nothing for their last stage of life.[10]

In fact, most people try to ignore signs that they are aging. Corinne, who lives in the same building as Maxine, quipped, "As far as aging goes, I try to avoid it." She added, "I am not concerned about it."

Burt, who is eighty-three, pronounced, "I am not eighty, I am seventy."

Frances, a former professor, told me that now her career is just maintenance of herself. As far as aging goes, she said, "When I turned eighty, I thought to myself, I am getting old. Now at eighty-six, I can say it out loud, 'I am old.'"

Sometime in this decade, no matter how strongly they have denied their aging in the past, people in their eighties finally come to terms with the fact that they are old, Once you admit you are old, some doors do close, but others open.

CONVERSATION STARTERS

- As a child, what kind of experiences did you have with people in their eighties?
- What stereotypes do you think most people have about older people?
- Now that you are in your eighties, how has your attitude about old people and aging changed?
- How has your life changed since you turned eighty?

TIPS FOR FAMILIES

- Talk with your eightysomething family member about the upsides of being in your eighties.
- Ask about who their role models of older people are and share with them your own.
- Find out what they miss most from when they were in their seventies and see if there is any way you can help them figure out some ways to address their issues.
- Remember that the most important thing you can do is to listen to your eightysomething—above all, old people do not want to be invisible and unheard.

CHAPTER 2

HEALTH MATTERS:
FIVE COPING STYLES

My husband, John, and I moved from our home on Independence Road to a retirement community when he was eighty-two and I was seventy-six. Since John had a number of health problems and wanted to move, it made sense to me. Yet I felt, but didn't say to him, I was *way* too young and healthy for a place that was populated with people who were mostly in their eighties. But I decided to be a good sport and to make the best of it.

The first night in our new community, as John and I made our way to the dining room, I was riveted by a parade of slow-moving people limping down the corridor. Each person, or so it seemed to me, was clutching a cane or was using a walker. The ancient riddle presented by the Sphinx to Oedipus came to mind and now, for the first time, actually made sense to me. *What walks on four legs in the morning, two legs at noon, and three legs in the evening?* Answer? Humans. Babies crawl on all fours, adults walk on two legs, and the elderly use a cane. I got it—canes are typical for the eightysomethings set—at least in a retirement community. The actual fact, I found out later, is somewhat less dramatic. Among all people in their eighties in the United States, only 33 percent of them have trouble walking.[1]

I thought, of course, people usually move into retirement homes when they have health problems. As we sat down at a table, I observed that there were many raised voices in the dining room. I soon became aware that most eightysomethings experience hearing loss. I had always thought that only a tiny fraction of people like my grandfather experienced hearing loss. Not so, it turns out. The actual data is over 66 percent of people in their eighties have hearing loss.[2] And while many of those with serious loss have hearing aids, a number don't use them. They insist that despite their outrageous price, they just don't work. It's true that the technology has been far from perfect.

Seven years later, my difficulties adjusting to living in the community are just a dim memory. Now it is home and feels like the right place for me to have a full and pleasant life. It was a wonderfully supportive place to be while my husband's health was failing and after he died. People gather around the grieving and surround them with care.

And, after seven years, I have aged and have developed some health issues myself. I take medicine for high blood pressure and a statin to keep my cholesterol down. My bladder leaks unpredictably but so far that is more of an annoyance than a major problem. I have lost much of my sense of taste and smell. A shame, but again, not truly a significant problem. And I learned that some loss of taste and smell is one of the common changes as people age into their eighties. But I can walk and hear, and only forget a word every now and then.

When I started interviewing for the book, I expected to find that all of those I interviewed would have many health problems. So, I was surprised that there was a sizable group of those whom I interviewed who, like me actually, had few or no health issues. This was one of my first "aha!" moments. Eightysomethings can be healthy. However, of course, most people in their eighties do have health issues. One of these eightysomethings summed up her life as "patch, patch, patch." And a whopping 52 percent of people in their eighties have four or more chronic conditions, according to the Consumer Reports National Research Center.[3] It is how they cope with their health issues that interests me most.

Doug, at eighty-six, is an example of a healthy man. He takes no prescription medicines at all. A former engineer, Doug and his wife have lived in the same house for over fifty years. Three years ago, one of his daughters and two small grandchildren moved in with them. He loves having them in the house and he happily helps out, taking one of the children to daycare each day. He admits that he has somewhat less energy nowadays, so he only goes on walks about twice a week. And he only skates a couple of times each winter. After telling me this, he commented, "I am almost embarrassed by my good fortune; I will probably fall apart all at once."

Hugh, eighty-eight, a Christian Scientist living in Connecticut, is another amazingly healthy person. A trim man, Hugh was wearing shorts the February day I interviewed him and he was just back from his daily walk. He told me that he has not been to the doctor since 1964. I must have looked shocked because he added quickly, apparently to reassure me, "I have been to the dentist though." When his wife died several years ago there was no funeral service and no mention of her death. He explained to me that she had just moved to another stage of life.

I couldn't help but wonder about the factors that explain Doug's and Hugh's amazing good health. Is it merely good genes and good luck? In Doug's case, I can't help but believe that being immersed in a multigenerational family where his help is needed contributes to his well-being. And for Hugh, I believe that his faith has much to do with his continued good health.

After interviewing many other eightysomethings who were less healthy, I discerned that people fall into five main groups according to how they cope with their health issues. Deniers, Stoics, Complainers, Worriers, and Realists. The coping style does not seem related to the severity of their health problems.

Deniers refuse to acknowledge their problems even when they are obvious to all those around them. They ignore chest pains and refuse to go to the doctor when they have shortness of breath. They continue to drive despite cataracts that should have been removed months before. They continue to eat quarts of ice cream despite their obesity. They drive their spouses and children crazy.

Andrew, eighty-eight, is a good example of a Denier. He is a small but intimidating man who was the CEO of a large company. He retired twenty-seven years ago. Five years ago, he was diagnosed with Parkinson's, and he and his wife moved to a retirement community in New Hampshire. His daily routine includes time in the wood working shop each morning. Despite his tremors, significant cognitive impairment, and tearful pleas from his wife, he refuses to stop using the power tools. He insists he is careful.

Unfortunately, it usually takes some kind of a calamity to get Deniers to pay attention to their bodies.

Stoics make up the largest group in my eightysomething sample. Stoics are like the literary character Pollyanna—remaining good-spirited and cheerful, even when they face situations that are painful and life-altering. At my retirement community, Stoics come to the dining room sporting bandages, crutches, and slings. As one woman said to me, "Why miss dinner just because you have a black eye and a large bandage around your head?" For these Stoics, it is definitely "stiff upper lip'" and "keep on moving." Regina and Cassy are both Stoics, and both have many serious health issues.

Regina, who was born in Italy, now lives with her husband of sixty-six years in a retirement community in upstate New York. She weighs a mere ninety-four pounds and takes dancing lessons three times a week. She mused, "I think the main reason I have lived so long, and am so healthy at eighty-four, is that I have taken care of my body. My mother was a nutrition nut. My whole childhood was her telling me 'eat this fish for your eyes, those carrots for memory.' I was given tonics and I survived typhoid as a child, so I must be a tough cookie. Today my hearing is not

so good and my heart has major electrical problems. Even so, I keep dancing and am very energetic."

Yes, Regina is a fine example of a Stoic. She knows she has health problems, but she minimizes them. I have a hunch that as long as she dances
she will survive for many more years.

Cassy, another example of a Stoic, is an eighty-seven-year-old diminutive woman with bright blue eyes and a radiant smile. She lives in New
York state, about a hundred miles from New York City. She told me,
"Everything changed for me in my eighties. I have had two hips replaced
and gotten two new knees. My arthritis is a problem. I have done the
falling thing, too, and was on a walker for several months. Now I can
walk just fine, but I have serious lung and breathing problems and
I've had skin cancer. Doctors' appointments keep me busy. Still I try to
exercise forty minutes a day and I can see just fine—that's a gift. I have
been so blessed." Cassy is so filled with joy and good spirits that she
had me believing she was okay despite the many issues she was dealing with.

Complainers are those who tell anyone who will listen about their back
pain, their acid reflux, their recent diarrhea, and on and on. This is an
extremely tiny group at my retirement community where complaining
about your health runs counter to the prevailing culture and puts you on
an imaginary black list where people may begin to shun you. It is okay,
however, to complain at length about the weather and the fact that the
chairs on the terrace are uncomfortable. Complainers are also a small
minority of those eightysomethings around the country whom I
interviewed.

Bunny, an eighty-five-year-old woman, is one of the Complainers. She
began our encounter with the proverbial organ recital: "Katharine, I am
having an awful time. My back aches all the time so I can't walk. I can't
eat anything that tastes good. My heartburn is horrible. My hearing is so
bad I really can't have a conversation. And now, my daughter has moved

to Colorado and left me high and dry. I can't believe she did that to me. I have no one to talk to now." It is hard to be empathic when there is a never-ending tale of woe. Her daughter told me when I interviewed her a few months later that it was quite a relief to be able to be out west.

Maud is one of the Worriers I spoke with. She lives in affordable housing in western Massachusetts. During our interview in her tiny apartment stuffed with furniture and artificial flowers, she told me, "I can hardly get up when I am on my knees and I worry about what I will do if it gets any worse. I stopped traveling because I was afraid I might get sick and, of course, I can't afford to travel, anyway. I don't go out often because I am afraid I might fall."

I know this type because my husband John was one of them. Although in public he appeared relaxed and carefree, in private, he was a Worrier. In his early eighties, when he was still fairly healthy, he worried about falling. So, he always walked with two hiking sticks to feel secure. He thought they made him look sporty rather than impaired. He worried about getting sick, so he took his blood pressure every day for years and would take to his bed with the slightest runny nose.

A short riff about falling. Almost all people in their eighties (except the Deniers) worry about falling. Eightysomethings hold onto the railings when going up and down stairs and rarely emerge out-of-doors if there is ice on the streets. And for good reason—because 40 percent of eightysomethings fall each year. Falls are the leading cause of fatal and non-fatal injuries in this age group. Everyone who is over eighty has a friend who has fallen and broken his or her hip and never really recovered. It is part of the culture of aging.

Lastly, we have the Realists. They are those wise souls who appropriately acknowledge their health conditions and their seriousness. They acknowledge their pain but don't dwell on it. They complain if it's bad. They pay attention to how their body feels and note changes and new symptoms. They go to the doctor and the dentist and they are not reckless. You do not have to second guess a Realist.

Ralph is a good example of a Realist. He is a tanned man with curly white hair. His energy level, however, is totally different from his ninety-year-old girlfriend's, as she continues to climb mountains and to ski. He spoke in a husky voice so softly that I had to keep asking him to repeat what he had said: "I had prostate cancer two years ago, needed an operation. Since then I have had urinary problems and sex with my girlfriend is not at all the way it was before the operation."

Ralph continued,

> After the cancer, then the next thing that happened was that my balance was off. I kept teetering around and banging into walls. It turned out I had fluid in my brain and I needed a shunt. The procedure has worked quite well and my brain seems okay. I also have neuropathy that has affected my feet. I take fourteen different kinds of medications each day and I can only walk about a block.
>
> We don't drink alcohol or eat red meat. Put bluntly, though, it's a lot of work. It's very tough. But each morning I wake up and say to myself I'm here, I am alive.

Some of the ways we cope depend on our ethnic background and culture. I recommend Monica McGoldrick's book, *Ethnicity and Family Therapy*, for anyone interested in pursuing this topic. For example, she explains that Irish people are likely to deny they have any pain while English are just stoic about the pain they feel. She has lots of fascinating material about how different groups experience and deal with health issues.

By the way, I see myself as a Stoic. My father didn't go to a doctor for thirty years. No one in my family got much attention for being sick, so as a child I didn't take to my bed or stay home if I felt a little off. As an adult I used to go to work when I was sick and several times my colleagues would take a look at me and send me home. Now in my eighties I like to think I am more sensible. I do go to the doctor much sooner now, but I probably still carry on a bit past the point that it is reasonable.

What else did I learn from my 128 interviews about eightysomethings and their health? First, I am convinced now that their attitude and usual coping style have more impact on their behavior than their actual health status. And most importantly, I observed that a decline in health in one's eighties is not always—in fact, is not usually—accompanied by a similar decline of good spirits. Many in their eighties feel happy—some happier than they have ever been before. This is the little-known fact about eightysomethings that we will explore and expand upon throughout this book.

Younger family members often have trouble understanding how their eightysomething relatives actually feel. They are sure they would be totally depressed if they had half the health issues that their eightysomething parent or relative is living with. Yet Cassy glows with joy and Ralph reports he has never been so happy in spite of how tough it is for him. Somewhere in the decade of their eighties, many people begin to see the glass half full. If they do not have dementia and are not in constant pain, eightysomethings count themselves lucky. They are able to take pleasure in what remains—they are alive.

CONVERSATION STARTERS
- How has your health changed since you turned eighty?
- How has this impacted your life?
- Do you believe you are a Denier, a Complainer, a Worrier, a Stoic, or a Realist in terms of your health? Explain.

- What are the positive things about your coping style?
- What are the downsides?

TIPS FOR FAMILIES

- If your parent is a Denier, you need to continue to bring their unacknowledged health issues to their attention even though they may not like it. Persist in getting them to the doctor if they are avoiding this.
- If your eightysomething is a Complainer, listen for a bit, but set a time limit. Remember you do not have to fix every complaint. Change the subject.
- For Worriers, reassure them in a calming way. Do not try to argue them out of their worry. Remind them that they tend to be overly pessimistic.
- For Stoics, self-care is the word. Explore with them specific actions they can take to care for themselves. Encourage them to notice how they are actually feeling.
- If your aging parent is a Realist, be aware that you are very lucky. Tell them how much you appreciate their good judgment.

CHAPTER 3

UPSIDE DOWN PARENTING

Most eightysomethings look at their family through the forgiving lens of love. Relegated to the back of their minds are the earlier disappointments about their kids and grandkids who never finished college, sons-in-laws that they would never have chosen for their beloved daughters, children who drink a bit too much, and those who are still finding themselves.

"My son is coming to visit on Friday," proclaimed Doris to the group of senior citizens gathered for "coffee and conversation" at a Council on Aging west of Boston. Doris, an eighty-four-year-old woman with bright orange hair and wearing a green baggy sweater, beamed. It was as if she had announced that royalty was arriving. The group smiled and nodded in recognition of the importance of this event for Doris.

Whenever Helga, an eighty-nine-year-old woman who lives in a retirement community in Seattle, meets someone new, she makes sure they know by the end of their conversation that she has five children, all of whom live nearby, and that she has eleven grandchildren. Helga feels she is definitely a winner in the game of life. Among eightysomethings, the competition about children and grandchildren is usually subtler. And besides, while numbers do count, one child, one grandchild, or even a niece or a godchild is enough for most eightysomethings to feel content.

When parents reach their eighties, a major shift typically takes place, turning upside down relationships in the family that have been constant for decades. As eightysomething parents become frailer and needier, their children step up and play an ever-increasing role in their day-to-day lives and their major decisions. In many ways, the adult children begin to act like parents of their own parents as they become more dependent and childlike.

In early childhood, parents are protectors, rule setters, authorities, and decision-makers. As children move into adulthood, they gain more and more autonomy, but the parent-child dynamic remains essentially intact. Adult children often continue to rely on their parents as a safety net. They look to their parents for a loan when they can't make ends meet and for help when buying a house. Even when adult children don't need material help from their parents, they often seek counsel from them about critical decisions such as a job change or a problem with a child.

Parents, as they age into their sixties and seventies, usually continue to operate almost independently. Somewhere along the way, though, a role reversal begins. Aging parents begin to need a little more help from their kids—to carry heavy objects, to set up a computer, to buy tickets online for an upcoming trip. As the years go by, children provide more and more assistance.

By the time their parents are in their eighties, the balance has shifted. Adult children have usually taken over hosting holiday dinners and managing family vacations. Most importantly, the children feel a new responsibility for their eightysomething parents' well-being. They go with their parents to medical appointments, help with their downsizing, and are involved in major decisions of all kinds. Often, they feel a new urgency to intervene when they have concerns about the parents.

Sometimes these shifts in the family dynamics happen easily and sometimes they are painful, as the stories of Milly, Cassy, Barbara, and Henry illustrate.

When Milly had a couple of fender benders in her early eighties, her three children urged her to stop driving. She told them, "Back off," and continued to drive as usual. Her son, Tim, repeatedly told her that he was afraid she would hurt someone. Milly ignored all his pleas and those of her other two children. One snowy day, when she was eighty-six, Milly smashed her car into the back of a school bus. At this point, the three children got together, and told her, "It's time. You are done driving." And it was. No fuss.

Eightysomethings like Millie, who behave in ways that are unsafe and put the lives of others at risk, pose a difficult challenge to their adult off-spring. There are no easy answers. The adult children are not sure when it is appropriate to take action and when they should let their aging parent make his or her own decision even if it seems like bad decision. What is their moral and civic responsibility? Can they take action without too much uproar? I got yet another perspective from a director of a senior center near Boston who told me, "We believe that old people have the right to make some decisions that may not be good for them. But it is hard to watch." As a psychotherapist, I have seen the necessity and bene-fits of intervening when it is a question of safety. But for many adult children limit setting with a parent is daunting if not almost impossible.

It was an easier transition for Cassy, whom we met in the previous chapter. She told me, "When there is a crisis now, my daughter is in charge." She continued, "When I fell on Christmas Eve, my daughter announced, 'We are going to the emergency room.' Of course, I didn't want to ruin the family holiday, but I did what she said. I can say 'no' at other times."

Barbara's story was a sad one. The day I interviewed her, Barbara was stylishly dressed with a big smile on her face but a slightly vacant look in her eyes. At eighty-six, she had moved a year earlier to a retirement com-munity. She told me how her daughter, Kara, helped her find the place and does a great deal for her. She visits every Wednesday and takes her to lunch. It was only at the very end of my interview that another side of the story emerged. Barbara confessed, still with a smile on her face, "I never told Kara that I didn't want to come here. And I don't ever want her to know how miserable I am here. I haven't made a single friend and am alone all day. But Kara has done so much for me I can't bear to hurt her."

Children of eightysomethings, like Barbara's daughter, Kara, are sometimes totally unaware of the feelings and inner thoughts of their apparently upbeat parent. They do not know just how cagey eightysomethings can be in concealing what is going on for them. Many of them not only hide their distress from their children, but they never talk to anybody about the problems they are having with such things as paying the bills or turning on their TVs. One doctor whose patients are mostly elderly told me, "You see what they let you see."

As an adult child, it takes asking some questions and observing one's parent closely to determine what their capabilities actually are. Several months after my interview with Barbara, I interviewed Kara. I learned from her that she had moved her mother to a Memory Care Facility. She admitted to me, "In retrospect, I should have moved her years before, because by the time she arrived at the retirement community, she didn't have the bandwidth to make any friends or even to find her way around."

The shift in parent/child relations was filled with bad feelings for Henry and his daughter Clare. Henry is a quiet and unassertive eighty-eight-year-old man living in his home of many years in the woods of New Hampshire. During our interview, Henry told me that for months he had been getting calls from Clare urging him to move to Arizona where she lived. She said she wanted to have him near her, so she could care for him. At first, the idea of sunny days all year sounded good to Henry. But when Clare put more pressure on him to move, Henry realized he did not want to leave his home and his town.

A few weeks later, Henry got a call from his doctor who told him that Clare had asked him to write a letter stating that Henry was no longer competent to make major decisions for himself. The doctor had refused to write such a letter but still Henry felt completely betrayed by what Clare had done. He came to feel that despite all Clare's protestations of love what she really wanted was to get control of his money. He was so upset that he would not talk to Clare for a year, and even now, two years later, their relationship remains chilly. Henry did tell me he is planning to move into town in the next year or so.

In Henry's case it is hard to tease apart all the factors. Is he still able to care for himself adequately or not? I couldn't tell, of course, whether Clare was after his money or just concerned for his well-being. I do know many adult children do worry: "Will my parents live so long that they burn up all my inheritance?" This issue is usually not discussed. I was unsettled when an adult child said to me in one interview, "I just wish my mother-in-law would die because we need the money for the kids' college."

In any case, I hope that Henry and Clare will begin to talk more—and more forthrightly. Severed relationships in a family are rarely the best solution.

Just to note here, elder abuse is a real problem. The most common form of abuse is financial mistreatment, followed by neglect, emotional mistreatment, physical mistreatment, and lastly sexual mistreatment. Perpetrators are most likely to be family members, then to be friends or neighbors, and then home aides.[1]

In many cases, eightysomethings do move closer to their families when they have lost a spouse or when they can no longer live independently. Moving closer means their adult child will not have to make numerous trips to deal with now predictable crises, and family will be close at hand if anything should happen. In short, they will be less of a burden on their child or children—the major worry of eightysomethings.

It is important to note that our culture values independence and self-reliance above everything else. Eightysomethings try desperately to avoid being dependent on anyone. In my view, they too often stay in their homes even when it means they are isolated and have few social contacts. Learning to be appropriately dependent, and to be interdependent, are perhaps better goals for the eightysomething set. But it is not an easy sell.

In other parts of the world, many people do not have resources to live alone and far away from neighbors. So they are less socially isolated.

The societal expectation that it is a daughter's responsibility to care for aging parents in need seems to be alive and well, old-fashioned as it may seem to some. But it is a fact that there is usually a big difference between the relationships of most daughters of eightysomethings and those of the sons.

For example, take Rosie, a divorced woman who is an accountant living in New Jersey. She told me she calls her mother in Buffalo every day, some days two or three times. Jim, Rosie's brother, calls their mom about once every other week. This gender difference is fairly typical. I once commented to a friend after hearing from none of my four sons for over a week, that, "As far as communication goes, four sons are about equal to one daughter."

When Rosie's mother moved to assisted living because of a chronic heart condition, Rosie didn't give up her job. But for over a decade, she flew from New Jersey to Buffalo once a month. She is lucky that she has a lot of flexibility in her work, so she can take long weekends to visit her mother. Many others, however, do not have the resources to make such visits to far-away parents.

The role reversal is never total. Margo, an eighty-seven-year-old mother of two daughters in their fifties, told me that, although her children have stepped up and are helping her more and more, she still is doing some parenting. One of her daughters, who is a single mom, is having a tough time. She gets depressed and is often overwhelmed. Margo finds herself providing a listening ear and ongoing counsel. It is a great comfort to her that she is still needed.

When aging eightysomethings are clearly in their final days, resistance to being dependent evaporates. Some people become totally childlike, entering what has been called a *second childhood*. They can no longer manage the tasks of daily life: walking, dressing, and eating. They may be incontinent and back in diapers. They cry more easily, and some become timid and clingy. They may regress to toddler ways like using only a spoon. When Virginia, my mother-in-law, was in the last month of her life, she would not eat anything except vanilla ice cream. I heard later this is not uncommon and it was explained to me by a nurse that vanilla ice cream is the food that is most like breast milk.

Children and parents remain central to each others' well-being through all the ups and downs of life. In the last weeks of my husband's life, when his world was getting smaller day by day, John would often say, "This was a great day. I talked with one of my sons." He didn't remember the details of the conversation but staying connected to his children and having me by his side, that was enough.

CONVERSATION STARTERS

- How have your relationships to family members shifted since you turned eighty?
- Has the process been smooth or bumpy? Explain.
- In what ways are you more dependent on your children or others than before? In what ways are you still independent?
- What is your attitude toward being more dependent? Do you feel annoyed? Resistant? Grateful? Accepting? Explain.

TIPS FOR FAMILIES

- One way to get started talking about a difficult topic with your eightysomething parent can go something like this: "I am wondering what it would be like for you to give up driving/to move/to get some help? How will you know it is the right time?" Listen to them first and then you can present your own views on the situation.

- Talk with your parent about what independence means to them and how important it is. Raise the importance of social connections for well-being.
- Eightysomethings like to be needed, to still do some parenting. So continue to ask for their advice or opinions.
- They also like to be useful—so at family occasions, give them the opportunity to help with a task rather than assuming they want to sit back and be served.
- Knowing that eightysomethings minimize their difficulties and often hide their problems from their children, take time to see for yourself if they can manage their bills, their phone, their schedule, etc. Find help for them if you find they need it.

CHAPTER 4

HOLDING ON AND LETTING GO

Author Florida Scott-Maxwell wrote, "Age puzzles me. I thought it was a quiet time. My seventies were interesting, and fairly serene, but my eighties are passionate. I grow more intense as I age. Inside we flame with a wild life that is almost incommunicable." She also wrote, "The crucial task of age is balance, a veritable tightrope of balance, just well enough, just brave enough . . ."[1]

The lifestyle of even the healthiest people in their eighties is different from when they were in their seventies. Each eightysomething must come to grips with losses. Typically, as they lose friends and family and as they experience decline in their physical capacity, they do feel they are retreating. It is a dance of both holding on and letting go. Joy and passion remain as well as sadness and anxiety.

My own story of holding on and letting go happened at the time when my husband was quite ill. I was struggling to do everything that I had always done—work, write, take care of John, and see my friends. I became tired and more tired, and then, I was exhausted. I felt like my inner gears were suddenly jamming. I forgot appointments, lost my keys and my purse. I felt disoriented and numb, almost like a robot, going mindlessly through my days.

At that point, I took a leave of absence from my psychotherapy practice and bowed out of all my commitments and regular activities and things went more smoothly. I realized that letting go was wise for me. But a year after John's death, when I was eighty-one, I had once again let myself get frantic and way too busy. Every now and then I would say to myself, "I really should let go of something." But I didn't. I kept on trying to do everything I used to do.

It was an encounter with a bird that summer that started my change. I was walking alone on a beach on a cold and windy day. I saw ahead of me a seagull standing alone in the sand, not moving. It had a huge bundle of greenish-brown, straw-like seaweed hanging from its mouth. "Drop it," I thought. And then, inexplicably, I heard myself say out loud, "You've got to let go of it." And as I heard my own voice, I realized I was talking to myself as well as the gull. I definitely had things that I needed to let go of, too.

A few days later I found myself walking into the office of my minister. I told her I would not be able to lead the six-session class on aging that I had previously agreed to facilitate. I was sorry, but knew it was the right thing for me to do. I then said "no" to being on a board that was trying to save a worthy organization. And then I let go of more activities that had become obligations drained of joy.

Slowly my numbness disappeared. But I knew myself well enough to know that I would eventually trick myself into saying "yes" to things I should say "no" to. I would have to keep on calling on that gull with its mouthful of seaweed for help. Letting go remains a challenge for me to this day.

Edith, Polly, Prescott, Vincent, Milton, and Maggie suggest the incredible range of the ways that eightysomethings are spending their days and how their pleasures change as they age. They show us, too, how eightysomethings deal with the wish to hold on and the need to let go.

They also demonstrate that many eightysomethings continue to do exciting things.

Edith, age eighty-one, a former English as a Second Language (ESL) teacher living in a college town in Indiana, is a whirlwind of activity. She has a windblown look about her with her gray hair going every which way. The day I met up with her she was outfitted in blue slacks, a yellow shirt, and a red sweater.

Edith told me, "I love being retired. I can do what I want, when I want. I am a wide person, not a deep one. There are very few things I am not interested in." And to prove her point, she told me she is a member of four book groups. She also edits a newsletter for her retirement community, serves on several committees, and sings in her church choir. Her husband died about six months before I interviewed her, and she told me with a little laugh that she feels guilty that she recovered so fast.

Edith admitted that what she doesn't like about aging are the physical restrictions. She added, "I largely ignore these age-related inevitabilities. I can't drive safely at night, but I keep postponing cataract surgery. I never go to the doctor. I did get hearing aids because I was annoying myself by saying, 'What?' way too often." She realizes she has some memory loss. It was frightening for her when she'd arrived at a meeting a few weeks before and discovered that she had completely forgotten that she was responsible for some tasks.

Edith continued, "I never have been one to be beset with worries. I did not worry when I took a trip recently and drove for nine hours all alone. I seem to worry a lot less about what others think of me than many other people. What has fallen away as I've gotten older is measuring myself against someone else. I do worry about underfunding for education, gun violence, and the political scene."

Edith needs to slow down and take stock. Probably she can still keep doing much of her present daily activities, but she can't do everything, as her own experience is beginning to teach her. But for people like her, this is never easy. She needs a wise guide to help her to become more realistic.

Polly, eighty-six, in contrast to Edith, leads a quiet life and has let go of many former pastimes and activities. A plump, short woman with sparkling blue eyes and a warm smile, Polly lives in the same town where she grew up. She married her high school boyfriend and they had five children in six years. All of them reside in the area and they are all in touch with her regularly. Two years ago she sold her small house and moved into an apartment. She explained, "The kids did it all." After the sale of the house, she was able to buy a new bedroom set and a new sofa. And then she sent a small check to each of the twelve grandchildren.

Although she doesn't do anything else at church the way she used to, Polly still goes to mass each week. She told me with a chuckle, "I just recently realized, I don't have to babysit anymore." She also doesn't go to the aerobics class that she attended for twenty-five years and she stopped her volunteer work when she was eighty-four. It was just too much. She falls asleep during movies now and doesn't follow the Red Sox anymore. She no longer travels, either. She is so glad she and a friend got a chance to see the Grand Canyon, Florida, and Ireland when she was in her sixties and seventies. She has made a group of new friends in the apartment. She laughed, saying, "I don't drink and I am the only one who can drive." But her holidays are always with family. Polly has let go of so many of these activities with apparent ease. She seems happy with her quieter lifestyle and at peace.

Prescott, age eighty, like Polly, leads a mostly sedentary life and like her, is also content. "I spend a lot of time on my front porch—surveying my property," said Prescott who lives in North Carolina with his wife and a grandson whom they adopted.

"As a black kid growing up in the south in a family of ten kids, joining the military was always my plan," he said. Prescott talks often with two of his sisters and his youngest brother and keeps in touch with most of the others now and then. After thirty years in the Air Force, Prescott worked for a couple of years, but never fully pursued another career: "Nowadays I don't do a whole lot. Get up and go to bed. My life is not full of anything. No going out at night. I do cut the grass. And my grandson is pretty much my responsibility."

Prescott explained that he has prostate cancer that has spread to his bones: "It jumped up and grabbed me. I go to the doctor every three months. I made it through the treatments. I feel all right and it doesn't get me down. I don't think about it much. I get tired and I have to rest a lot."

He continued: "I watch a lot of TV sports, a lot of surfing through the channels. I am not much of a reader, but I think it's important to know what's going on and voting is always important. There is not much encouraging going on. I play solitaire every day on my iPad. I like it; you play the game and then you move on to the next thing. I like the same stuff forever. I don't need to do a whole lot of changing." Prescott has let go of many of his former activities and made his peace with his limitations. He is not striving to accomplish more, and he accepts his situation with equanimity.

Vincent, eighty-eight, a sallow, wrinkled man, with no resources except Medicaid, lives at a nursing home. He is one who rages against his present circumstances. In the first five minutes of our time together, he told me, "I don't do a damn thing. I don't know if I am better off dead or alive. I am not happy here. I am an old-time smoker and you can't even smoke here; it's terrible. The food here is terrible. I don't eat any meat here, I just eat potatoes. That's all I eat. And the little tangerines they have for dessert. My weight is down to nothing. And my roommate is terrible, he bangs on his chair all the time and during the night he growls."

Vincent went on to tell me that he has six daughters. "I am going to be honest and tell you that a couple don't even talk to me," he said. "My sister doesn't talk to me either. You never would have seen my father or mother in a place like this. The kids took them in. I have a grandson and he's been saying he'll come for a month, but I haven't seen him. I took him to Chinatown and taught him to drive. It's pretty sad. I am not sure how long I am going to last."

Still Vincent has his small pleasures: "I play bingo and I like it—something to do. A trip to the doctor is a day out of here. I smoke my cigarette in the car and I am happy as hell." Anger can be energizing, and Vincent's rage is part of what keeps him going. But it is too bad for him that he has let so many of his relationships with his family stay broken.

Unlike Vincent, Milton, eighty-eight, who lives in southern California, is a husky, healthy-looking man who is contented with his life. Milton tells me with pride that he is doing just about what he has always done for the last twenty years. Here is how he describes his routine: "I swim five times a week and go to the gym on the other days. I noticed in the last couple of months, however, that I am not quite as fast as I used to be when I swim. I used to do a lap in ninety seconds and now it takes me ninety-five. I socialize in the sauna after exercising, but basically I am a loner. I cook my own meals, watch the salt, the fat, the carbs. I have four different meals that I cook, and I make a different one each week. I do seem to tire more easily and move more slowly than I used to."

When I asked Milton about a high point in the last year, a time he particularly enjoyed, he was stumped. Finally, he came up with an answer: "I went for my annual physical and my doctor told me I was in the top one half of one percent of his patients in terms of my health. He said I had the body of a seventy-year-old. That made me very happy, that was a great moment."

What struck me most was how tightly Milton is holding on to his routines and how satisfied he was with his aloneness. He is one that insists he doesn't need other people. He broke up with his girlfriend and is angry with his son. Life seems to be working well for him currently, but I wonder how he will fare once his rigorous schedule is no longer possible.

Maggie has also, like Milton, made unusual choices that suit her but would not be everybody's cup of tea. Eighty-eight years old, she lives alone in an old farmhouse out in the countryside in upstate New York five miles from town. Like all the others I interviewed, her life today is a combination of holding on and letting go. She is holding on to her house. She said she and her house are partners and she wants to stay there despite the inconveniences: "I love being in the country—looking out the window and seeing a wild turkey or a porcupine on a branch of my apple tree. I enjoy the silence."

She continued, "But I took the car keys away from myself and this changed my life. It was the car's fault," she added wryly. "A van takes me to the doctor." Maggie has also held on to directing plays several times a year at the nearby community theater. This year she directed *As You Like It*. She said, "When I am doing a play I check in with my inner voice, that has got to be the guiding thing. And I am writing some poetry.

"My whole day is a challenge, though, and takes courage," she admitted. "Just to get going takes me three hours. With my arthritis everything takes me so long." She showed me her hands that are gnarled like an ancient bonsai tree. As I looked at her hands and baggy, dark green pants and T-shirt, I can't imagine how she is able to get dressed by herself. She explained, "I go into patience gear."

After dressing, she meditates, watching her breaths come in and out. And then she prays—"for people, my children, my grandchildren, to be mindful, thankful, joyful, to remember." She said, "I am trying to let go of my puny plans and go with what's there—another person or a situation. It's work to accept limitations, as you get old."

My interview with Maggie reminded me of a beautiful passage about the last stage of life in *King Lear*. Lear says to his beloved daughter Cordelia:

> Come, let's away to prison:
> We two alone will sing like birds i'the cage:
> When thou dost ask me blessing, I'll kneel down
> And ask of thee forgiveness: so we'll live,
> And pray and sing and tell old tales, and laugh
> At gilded butterflies.[2]

Several things are noteworthy about the passage. First, physical limitations for some people in their eighties, can make daily life a kind of prison. For many, there comes a time when being productive in the usual ways is just no longer possible. Doing is almost impossible. Shakespeare suggests that praying, singing, storytelling, and laughing are the rightful activities of that last stage of life. None of these activities have any purpose or produce anything. But they all can bring great meaning to life, suggests Helen Luke, a Jungian analyst, who has written a wonderful book, *Old Age*. It was she who first drew my attention to this passage in *Lear*.

Maggie has learned how to hold on to what matters most to her, whether it is totally rational or not, and to let go of other things, especially when it would be unsafe or foolish not to. She also positively enjoys *not doing*. She prizes the silence and just being. She has reinvented her life with her poetry, her plays, and her prayers.

All eightysomethings deal with their aging in their own way. Vincent is angry but has his pleasures, Edith and Milton strive to keep doing everything as always, while Polly and Prescott have let go of many activities and yet are content. Many in their eighties are *doing* things they find exciting. (See Appendix I.) From Maggie, but also from many of the others whom I interviewed, I became aware of a new possibility for all of us, an unanticipated final flowering in old age, a time of *being* and inner peace.

CONVERSATION STARTERS

- Which activities have you held onto in your eighties? How is that for you?
- What have you let go of and what has been your attitude about letting go? Sadness? Frustration? Conflict? No big deal? Relief?

- What role do singing, praying, laughing, and storytelling have in your life now?
- What are your pleasures?

TIPS FOR FAMILIES

- You may get impatient with how long it takes eightysomethings to do ordinary tasks like getting dressed. It is helpful if you are able to go into patience mode and slow yourself down. Eightysomethings are slow.
- Take time to hear stories about your eightysomething's life. Just listen.
- Your aging relative may need encouragement to stop doing so much—cooking, caring for grandchildren, volunteering. Give them your permission to let go of these activities. It is their turn to enjoy just being.
- Figure out ways to help your eightysomething get more of their small pleasures.

CHAPTER 5

FRIENDS

There are many benefits to having friends throughout life, but they are especially important for older people. Friends not only improve the quality of life of older people by bringing joy and fun, but they also prolong life by lowering the risk of dementia, boosting the immune system, and encouraging healthy behaviors. A recent study by William Chopik, a social psychologist at Michigan State University who studies how relationships change over time, came to an interesting additional finding: having good friends is even more important than family relationships in determining how happy older people feel.[1]

Friendships of people who are in their eighties are different, however, from earlier times in their lives because many in their age cohort have already died. And because their lifestyles are different than before. In addition, friendship is different for men and for women throughout their lives.

Almost every man whom I interviewed told me that as an adult he had few or no friends at all. Or he said that his wife was his best friend and often his only friend. While he might play golf or watch sporting events with other men, he didn't really talk about anything personal with them. For these men, then, nothing much changes when they age into their eighties. They continue to have no friends.

Most men, if their wife dies before they do, feel completely at sea. Not only have they lost their wife and their best friend, but, in addition, their wife has been in charge of running the house, their social life as a couple, and maintaining family relationships. Many men have little experience in setting up get-togethers and reaching out to others.

When a wife dies, some men within a surprisingly short time—sometimes even within mere weeks—find a new companion. Some join grief or support groups. Often these are places where they meet their new companion. Other men seek out the company of men, like Dale, for example, who lives in a retirement community near Philadelphia. He began attending a breakfast group of about ten men each morning. He feels it is a nice to have some time with just guys because their community has so many women.

There are exceptions, of course, to this picture of the friendless male. Take Sam, who is eighty-three and lives in New York with a nephew. He left Alabama and went north to get a degree in guidance counseling in Michigan. He still smarts at being accused of plagiarism by a professor who could not believe a black man from Alabama could write an outstanding paper. He was a counselor for thirty years, retiring when he was sixty.

Sam never married, but he has never been lonely because he is in touch with friends and his siblings—four sisters and two brothers: "People want to be my friend. I am still in touch with at least fifty of them. Each month I make out an itinerary to figure out my schedule."

I was quite surprised when Sam went on to tell me how he spends his time. "Every day I am out of the apartment by noon and I spend a few hours shooting pool with some friends," he said. "Then I go bar hopping. I don't join clubs or organizations—and I am not a church person. I have my own schedule, and no one tells me what to do. I am a happy man."

Ward, who is eighty-one and lives in northern California at a retirement village, is another eightysomething man with an unusually large number of friends. He, rather than his wife, is almost always the one to suggest inviting friends to sit with them at dinner, but he gets his wife to make the calls. Last summer, Ward and his wife and their two dogs headed for the east coast in their RV. They took six weeks to make the trip, stopping to see more than a dozen old friends along the way. Back at home, Ward attends several groups, including a ROMEO group—retired old men eating out—that meets once a week for lunch and a book group.

For most women, unlike so many men, friends have always been hugely important. What changes for them in their eighties is that friends become even more important—especially if their husband has died, which is so often the case. There are many more widows than widowers among eightysomethings because women, of course, live on average about five years longer than men. And also, because women frequently married men who were a few years older than they were. Double jeopardy. And, of course, many of their women friends have died as well.

Women usually keep on making new friends. But they differ in their skills in making friends and their motivation to do so. Dot, Mary Elizabeth, Pamela, and Laurel illustrate the many faces of friendship for eightysomething women.

Dot, eighty-two, is one who has figured out how to keep making friends. I met up with her at a senior center in a small city in western Massachusetts. She had straight white hair and a strong angular face and was wearing jeans and sensible brown shoes. She began, "Most of my friends have died and I live alone in a condo."

"For years," Dot continued, "I was in a group of six women who played canasta ever week. Most of them are gone now. When they started passing, we got the husbands to fill in. But now they are gone, too, so I play Scrabble with two new friends. And I come here to the senior center for company. Now that I am in my eighties, I just love my life. It all gets very easy and pleasant."

I am impressed by the continuing adaptations that Dot has made to the losses of her friends—bringing in the husbands as some of the women died and then switching to Scrabble. What a good metaphor for how to thrive in your eighties. You need to keep playing, but you may have to accept playing with new people and even be ready to change what game you play as your situation evolves.

Mary Elizabeth, eighty-two, has not been as successful as Dot as far as friendship goes. Mary Elizabeth, who is overweight and a smoker, admits, "I am a recluse. Most people I know are married or they have died. I don't have money and that makes it hard because my friends can do more things than I can afford and can travel. I have had to fend for myself but, basically, I just hole up. I can't read with my macular degeneration and that means I can't volunteer. Actually, I am joined at the hip to my iPad."

Mary Elizabeth is unhappy about her isolation but seems to blame it on her financial situation. She does not seem to acknowledge that she has any control over how her life is playing out. What a shame, I thought, as we wound up our conversation, and how much she could benefit from a group of some kind.

Pamela, eighty-eight, unlike Mary Elizabeth, is far from isolated. She has been a widow for fifteen years and has a lived in a retirement community for the last twelve. Pamela, with lovely golden hair, the air of a former beauty, and a bad limp from a hip operation that turned out poorly, told me, "My good friends have mostly died—just this week I learned about two more friends from college who have died. I have made lots of new friends over the last years." But she continued, "I am not looking for intimacy. I had such a wonderful marriage that my marriage continues to sustain me." She added, "I don't believe in best friends. I don't find it necessary to talk about my children all the time like some people here and I am not lonely. When I see someone who seems lonely, I often invite them to have dinner with me." She is another person who has successfully adapted to her changing circumstances. She has created the situation that she wants.

Laurel, a black woman who lives in Albuquerque in an apartment with her sister, told me, "I have found this stage the very best. I have time to do things, time to enjoy my friends, to enjoy being. Many friends have passed, so I have maybe nine or ten friends today. We have lunch, have spa days, go out to dinner. We no longer do the self-improvement stuff we used to and I don't believe it is necessary to do physical exercise."

Laurel continued, "At eighty-five, I see myself in the fourth stage of life, that is, the winter of life—a time of peace and wisdom. Every morning I say a number of affirmations such as, 'I will view everything that the universe sets before me with love and appreciation.' And I am grateful that I always have enough money to share with my family. I see my job to become love."

I learned that not all women are as filled with love and peace as Laurel; there are a few "mean girls" among eightysomethings who can make a retirement community feel like middle school all over again, as Ethel and Denise found out. Ethel, eighty-nine, is a Complainer. I interviewed both Ethel and her daughter, Ashleigh. Ashleigh is upset by how her mom is getting treated at the assisted living facility to which she recently moved. "When anyone ventures within six feet of Ethel," Ashleigh explained, "she begins monologuing in a loud voice about everything that is wrong with the facility. People drift away quickly. When she goes to sit down at a table at dinner where there are a few empty places, those sitting at the table usually tell her, 'We are saving those places for other people.'" Ethel tells Ashleigh that she knows that isn't really true and it makes her feel terrible. Ashleigh is upset, too, but she told me, "I understand all too well just how difficult my mom is."

Denise is another woman who has met up with some "mean girls." She lives in affordable housing for the elderly in a small town. She told me,

> When I moved in, I got bullied. A couple of the women snubbed me and told everyone else I didn't have any friends. Yes, it's true that I was too busy to have coffee and I do think different from them. Then when I planted some flowers they said, "Who told you that you can plant flowers?" My feelings were hurt. When I used the washing machine on Wednesday, they told me, "You can't wash on Wednesdays." It was awful. I wasn't doing anything. It took two years for them to leave me alone. The office took care of it.

Denise says she still doesn't have any friends, but no one bothers her now.

Then there are those eightysomethings, like Elena, whose best friend is their pet. Elena, eighty-three, is from Brazil and lives in Illinois in a retirement community. As she has aged, her English, which was once fairly fluent, is getting worse each year. Elena got a dog from a friend about six months before I interviewed her. She told me, "Every day I walk him. He gives me the activity I missed. He goes everywhere with me. I talk to him in Portuguese. He is so cute. I put the music on and dance with him. I used to take him when I got my food in the dining room, but people complained because he barked, and I had to stop. I love that dog so much. He changed my life."

My own experience of making new friends in my eighties came as my husband's health was failing and he needed to go on dialysis. I had friends, but I realized I needed more support for this difficult time. I called two acquaintances in my retirement community, Peter and Carol, whose spouses were also very sick. Peter's wife had advanced dementia and Carol's husband with Parkinson's disease was dying. Before long we were getting together once a week to talk about all that we were going through. Week after week we talked about the ups and downs of our lives and how we were faring. At times we mourned our losses and we encouraged each other to take care of ourselves. A year later both husbands had died, Peter's wife had moved to the memory unit, and we were still talking about our grief.

One day, one of us came up with a shocking thought. "You know, we could do something fun—the three of us could go to Sonoma or Mexico or Florida or even Greece." Gradually the idea of a trip became more than a fantasy and we called a travel agent. And a few months later, the three of us flew off to Puerto Rico for six days at a seaside resort. We were an odd trio, two women and one man, the man using a walker. None of us were married or related to each other. "Just friends," we said over and over. Clearly three eightysomething friends traveling for fun, and having fun, was an unusual sight.

That trip was a turning point for me. I realized once again that I could be proactive and make more choices about my life. Even though I was still grieving the loss of John, even though I was eighty-two, I could make new friends, take a trip, and enjoy myself.

As I thought about what I had learned about friends and friendship from my interviews, it occurred to me that we all need three different kinds of friends to really thrive. First, we need friends who can provide practical help when we need it. Second, we need friends with whom we can talk honestly about our feelings and explore what is really going on for us. Lastly, we need friends who are fun to be with and who we can do things with.

For eightysomethings, dealing with losses becomes a central task. We all need to find a way to acknowledge our losses, express our feelings, to grieve. But it is also important to be able to move on, to have the strength to keep on connecting with people and making new friends. While new friends can never replace relationships of decades or a lifetime, we humans are social beings. We need connections to thrive.

For some people, like Barbara and Denise, this may be almost impossible. Many of us do not know how to grieve. Some people think they do just fine without other people. And some people, especially introverts, are truly happy with far fewer friends and social engagement than others. Some people in their eighties have disabilities or living situations that truly make social engagement just too difficult. And it is important to remember that we all have the right to make choices that may not be the wisest. But the main point is that having friends brings happiness throughout life, and especially when one is an eightysomething.

My interviews reaffirmed what I knew already as a social psychologist, too. Participating in groups and community organizations and continuing to attend religious services provide useful support systems for people in their eighties. Often by the time they are eighty, however, many people avoid taking on roles with significant responsibilities. They relish being able to use their advanced age as an excuse to beg off. But just by attending a group or going to a meeting, there are immense benefits to older people. Getting out and seeing people is stimulating to the brain and usually energizing.

Eightysomethings do not have to attend committees or be active in formal organizations to thrive. But until they are actively dying, they do need to find a way that suits them to stay engaged in life and connected to some other people. This need doesn't change when we turn eighty; it becomes even more urgent.

CONVERSATION STARTERS

- What has been the role of friendship in your eighties?
- Do you now have all three types of friends—those who can help you, those you can share your thoughts with, and those you can do things with? Say more about that.
- Have you made some new friends in your eighties and how did that happen?
- What groups and organizations are part of your regular schedule and what do like about each of them?

TIPS FOR FAMILIES

- Talk about friends and friendship. Just listening is helpful. Ask about loneliness, too.
- Encourage your eightysomething to continue with the activities that have meant something to them over the years. Help them stop going to activities they really don't like.
- Help your eightysomething figure out how they can continue to connect with old friends.
- Discuss people they know whom they would like to get to know better. Explore their experience reaching out to friends and what that is like for them.

CHAPTER 6

LOVE AND SEX

"This time there will be no honeymoon," said Chaya, eighty-five, a widow with dyed red hair, piercing black eyes, and several double chins living in upstate New York. The groom, Miles, is an old family friend, she explained, "He is very energetic, pretty successful, an engineer and still working. It is so nice to have somebody there for you. He does talk a lot more than he did before. When he goes on and on I say, 'Cut it short.' Not very nice. He is also very overweight and loves to eat. That is my biggest problem. But I count my blessings."

She continued:

> I am really in love with him. The heart is still twenty though
> you are not seventeen any more. The feeling is still the same.
> Never in my wildest dreams did I think I would marry again.
> Actually I have missed the companionship, the touching, too.
> My first husband died of cancer when he was only forty-seven
> and I was on my own, a single mom with two daughters, for
> fifteen years. I married again in my sixties and was, sadly, wid-
> owed a second time four years ago.
>
> Two years ago, Miles calls me up out of the blue. His wife has
> died, and he asks, "Can I come and visit you?" So he comes from
> New Jersey to see me here and after a just few visits, he tells me,
> "I don't want to be alone any longer. You know my kids, you
> know my friends, I want to marry you. We can keep both places."

As Chaya's story suggests, the desire for love and intimacy does not diminish with age. Most eightysomethings, like most other people, yearn for a relationship with emotional closeness, physical touching, and sometimes sex. Studies have shown that many people with health problems, depression, and cognitive issues seek a close relationship. But how we love when we are in the eighties is different from when we were young. Chaya is quite realistic about Miles's shortcomings and is still able to love him. She has put away the rose-colored glasses.

In the United States, however, there is still a commonly held assumption that sex is only for the young. For many people, the idea of old people, like eightysomethings, having sex is gross or weird. Any elderly man who is interested in sex is a "dirty old man." Many people in the past believed that women were supposed to be sexless after they reached sixty. Judith Viorst wrote in 1986, "The old often live half-lives, because they know they would arouse disgust and fear if they attempted to live whole ones."[1]

These puritanical attitudes have been modified in recent years. Today, the fact that we are sexual beings and we are interested in sex our whole lives is more widely accepted. The benefits of sex have also been acknowledged; sex improves overall health and improves self-esteem. According to a 2015 study, 29 percent of men in their eighties and 25 percent of women in their eighties are sexually active.[2]

The policies at the Hebrew Home at Riverdale, a nursing home in the Bronx, reflects this more enlightened perspective. The Hebrew Home has an explicit sexual expression policy that allows for privacy among patients. They can close the door to their room and have time without staff interruptions. The administration encourages new relationships among patients by sponsoring their own dating service and hosting a senior prom.[3]

The frequency of sex does inevitably decline over time for reasons other than the ageist attitudes about older people and sex. Multiple health issues can create challenges for sexual activity for couples in their eighties. The majority of men in their eighties report erectile difficulties; the number of jokes about Viagra that circulate among men in some retirement communities speaks to the prevalence of the issue. Jack, who is a retired doctor living in a retirement community in southern California, shared with me his observation about sex in one's eighties, "There are few one night stands among eightysomethings. It is all about intimacy."

Women mentioned problems with getting aroused and having orgasms, but there is research that eightysomething women have the highest levels of satisfaction with their sexual life compared to other older age groups.[4] This may, I believe, reflect less about the actual sex that is taking place and more about the gratitude that comes in your eighties when you have a partner, especially since so many others are alone.

In terms of eightysomethings' attitudes and sexual activity, I have identified four groups:

1. Those who are not interested in sex;
2. Those who remain interested in sex but are without a partner;
3. Those who have partners who are interested in sex but who are struggling to adapt to their changing circumstances, and, finally;
4. Those with partners who report they are happy with the sexual activity and intimacy that they have.

First, the not-interested-in-sex. A large proportion of people in their eighties report that they are not sexually active and many of them say they couldn't care less about it at this point in their lives. A woman I interviewed pronounced with great authority, "People in their eighties don't care about that." For her, sex was in the past. But she was wrong in assuming that everyone else is as uninterested in sex as she is.

Next are those eightysomethings who are without a partner and who report how much they miss their partner—the touching, the talking, the cuddling, the sex—all of it. Some of them told me that they can go through a whole week and not be touched by anyone. How sad and lonely they are. Others of these now-singles have found ways to touch and be touched. They get massages. One woman told me she looks forward to going to the hair salon. The touching that comes with having her hair washed feels so soothing. Then there are the pets—dogs and cats—to stroke and pet. What can feel more cozy and comforting than sitting with a cat in your lap as you watch television? And the grandchildren, since it is usually okay for a grandparent to hug and squeeze a grandchild, even a huge teenager. One of those I interviewed told me, "Of course, there is always masturbation." Others told me that masturbation was never part of their personal experience and to this day they have not ever even said the word out loud.

The third group of eightysomethings consists of partners who have issues about sex of one sort or another. They may have different levels of desire and interest as well as differing capabilities to be sexually active. In the eighties, as reported earlier in the chapter, the majority of men experience erectile dysfunction. Some men turn to Viagra or other prescription drugs, although among those I interviewed, it didn't really work for them. After the failure of Viagra or after a new disability arrives, many couples give up all sexual activity. Several women told me they were afraid to say anything that might make their partner feel bad or hurt his pride. Couples who have never talked about sex find it difficult to learn how to do so in their eighties. This is too bad, because talking about what is happening could be so helpful. Of course, some couples do adapt. They figure out ways to give pleasure to each other besides intercourse.

The last group are those partners who continue to be happily intimate in many ways with or without intercourse. One man said to me how lucky he feels every day when he wakes up and he has a partner to hold him. He and his wife know this togetherness can't last forever; but they have learned not to worry about the future and not to focus on what is missing. They will enjoy this day.

Lorna, eighty-five, is another person who is grateful every day for Judd, her partner of the last twenty-six years. Both of them have serious health issues, so much of their loving relationship is about caretaking. It is a second marriage for them both and between them they have eight children. Their two families have blended well and they celebrate holidays together.

Lorna is a diminutive dynamo with a pixie hairdo, who, at four feet eleven, is a bundle of energy. Retired for years, Lorna works diligently on a couple of committees to raise money for special projects at the local high school and for disaster relief. And Judd is active, too.

Lorna and Judd also have multiple health problems. "We have Rule Number One," said Lorna with a chuckle, "One of us has to be okay at all times." They have what they call "sweet days" on Thursdays when they don't schedule any outside activities and they just hang out together. "Some Thursdays we never get out of our pajamas. We are so happy and so blessed."

Of course, not all eightysomething marriages are happy. Take Vicki and Don. Vicki, at eighty-six, looked to me like a faded cheerleader. She told me that their marriage has been "rocky" for decades: "I have more friends than Don and we go our separate ways most of the time." Don, she said, turned out to be a misfit in business. He changed jobs often and lost most of their money several times. Now their budget is very tight and their small pension is not enough.

They live in a very small house and Vicki is not sure how long they can hold on to it. She rarely sees their grandchildren because they all live far away, and they don't have money for travel. "I'd love to go to New York and Jerusalem, too, but you can't do everything you thought you would," she said. "I can't help but wonder what would have happened if we had split years ago."

And, although it is extremely rare, some long-term marriages fall apart. Kitty, a chic woman with a house full of art from Haiti and Guatemala, kept up a good front giving parties and entertaining her neighborhood. Still, at her fiftieth anniversary party there were jokes about how unsuited Kitty and her husband Chandler were to each other. Soon after that party, at a college reunion, Kitty met Bob, a widower, who was eighty-two at the time. Kitty said it was love at first sight. After a year of emails and phone calls, Kitty separated from Chandler. Now, three years later, Kitty and Bob live together but have decided not to marry. Kitty said it is basically because of financial issues that they won't marry.

A footnote on the Kitty and Chandler story. Chandler refuses to meet Bob or go to family events like the graduations of their grandchildren if Bob will be there. He said it is because "Kitty is living in sin." And Kitty's daughter found the divorce of her parents very difficult even though she was in her fifties. Love and divorce are complicated at every age.

Back to the decision not to marry. This stance is typical of most new eightysomethings couples. The financial issues, whether the couples are rich or poor, are usually the most important factors. The health issues, the uncertainty of the future, and unenthusiastic children all come into play. As my twice-divorced friend, Rosie, who has had the same boyfriend for thirty years, said to me, "Why get married, what's the point?" In my retirement community, with a number of recently-formed couples, there has only been one wedding in the last fifteen years. At a retirement community in southern California of about five hundred residents one of those I talked with reported that seventeen new couples had gotten together over the last ten years. None had married, though some moved in together. Most eightysomethings continue to live alone but they feel happy when they see a new romance unfolding before their eyes.

For eightysomethings who are gay, it can be more difficult. They have lived through times when there were great pressures to remain in the closet. At my retirement community, for example, there are no openly gay people. But with the constant flow of stories about LGBTQ issues in the media, this will probably change in the near future. And it is not too surprising that there are a few people in their eighties, like Frank, who have chosen to come out.

Frank, at eighty-five, is movie-star-handsome with ruddy cheeks and a full head of salt and pepper hair. He told his family that he was gay just a year ago:

> I am happier, healthier than I have ever been. I didn't come out for eighty-four years because of ignorance, guilt, and shame. So last summer at a family picnic, I screwed up my courage and told my kids and their spouses, "I am gay." The sky did not fall—we just talked. My daughter did say to her husband, "Now, don't you get any ideas." And my family is still talking to me. No, I don't have a partner. About coming out, I had to do it. A great burden left my heart. I don't have any secrets any more.

But life is never simple. When I interviewed Frank's daughter who was at that family gathering when he came out, she told me how angry she is at her dad, "I can't believe it, he was lying to me my whole life." I understand her being upset. Still I hope she can begin to look at her father with more compassion.

But the main story of love and sex and eightysomethings is about the 60 percent who are single. Many of these are widows and widowers, but it also includes those never married and the divorced. All of their stories are unique, although there are some patterns that can be discerned.

Take Myra, eighty-six, who remains focused on her husband of sixty years who died suddenly of a heart attack eight years ago. She is typical of a group of women and men whose energy and thoughts remain with their beloved spouse, often forever. Myra, a calm, willowy woman whose white hair is swept into a bun, told me, "I feel like I am half a person and like I will be just putting in time for the rest of my life. I hurt the whole time. It is still a shock to be alone—nobody breathing next to me, nobody to cook for, nobody to eat with, and no one to chat with."

Myra spoke so softly that I missed some of what she said. When I asked her to speak louder, she didn't seem able to raise her voice. I strained to catch her words. As a psychologist, I asked myself what the small voice is about—is it a medical issue? Or does it reflect her unremitting sadness?

Two years ago Myra had a heart attack herself, but she has recovered well. Her two sons living in neighboring towns help her with her finances and accompany her to her heart specialist. She remains active, volunteering one day a week at the library and spending many hours in the spring and summer in her garden. She said, "I just can't bear to sell the house. I dread living into my nineties—I don't want to live to be ninety-six and be in a wheel chair like my uncle." As our interview came to an end I became aware that I had started feeling sad myself, because she was so heartbroken and because the future is so bleak for her and because emotions are contagious. While this attitude is not common, there is a small minority of people who are unable to move forward with their life. What helps is often getting involved with the grandchildren, joining a support group, or moving to a retirement community.

Most of those who are widows and widowers in their eighties, like Myra, do remain single. But eventually, most of them find some of the closeness they want from others. They spend more time with their siblings and their friends. They lean on their children and especially their daughters. They connect with grandchildren, nieces, and nephews.

And, as we have seen, some eightysomethings, after grieving for months or years for their spouse, find another companion. Stan, a widower, whom I interviewed at a senior center west of Boston, glowed as he told me that he had a new girlfriend. She is eighty-three and he is eighty-four. As he left, he shyly handed me a piece of paper, saying, "You might like this for your book, love prevails."

A Senior's Solace

Who could have possibly known
After all that life had shown
My wife, my love has passed
Fond memories and offspring will last
With most of my life behind me
A brand new world would find me
When first I saw her I couldn't resist
From letting her know that I exist
Over coffee we shared our thought and schemes
And soon there was love invading our dreams
And much to our complete surprise
The loneliness finally left our eyes
"It ain't over til it's over," said a wise man then
"It's like déjà vu all over again"
So embrace and nurture all the joys you see
Before time makes us history

—*Anonymous*

This poem catches the pathos of love in the eighties, a love sandwiched between the long past and a limited future. I didn't get to ask him where he found this poem.

Now, to my own story of love as an eightysomething. One day out of the blue, when I had been a widow for a year, I received a letter from Michael, a classmate of mine from elementary school who was living in

Connecticut. He suggested lunch in Boston. I had not seen him since we were eleven; we were now eighty-two. But I had never forgotten that when we were in fourth grade Michael had told me once that he liked me. Michael was a psychologist like me, although he was now retired and spent his time painting watercolors. The sense of familiarity, coming from many years spent in the same classroom, cast a golden haze over the lunch. Michael told me he was looking for someone to move in with him.

Soon Michael and I were meeting halfway between our towns for lunch. I found Michael empathic and reliable. It seemed easy. By late spring, I was spending weekends at Michael's house by the sea. We walked on the beach, went out to restaurants, and watched TV. I told my friends and my family about my new boyfriend.

But there were some dark clouds in this picture. Michael was a loner with no real friends and little need to chat. My time with him began to feel uncomfortable. He said that he wanted a partner who would move to his house. I realized I wasn't attracted to him and didn't want to be Michael's partner or even to spend much time with him. And so it unraveled rather quickly. When we officially broke up, I felt enormous relief. This was followed by regret that I got involved so quickly with someone so ill-suited to me.

That's how I learned, firsthand, that love in one's eighties has all the complications of youthful relationships and more. There are always the universal issues of commitment and compatibility but add to that lifestyles and habits that have been honed over a lifetime as well as health issues.

And so, like most other eightysomethings, I found myself back in the ranks of the singles who are free from responsibilities for others. But, also, back to the loneliness of life without a partner.

As the months went by, I began having dinner more often with Peter, who had been part of my support group for the last three years. Gradually, as more months went by, Peter and I realized that we were more than friends and that we had become a couple. At the astonishing age of eighty-four, I had a new love.

CONVERSATION STARTERS

- Have you heard negative comments about older people having sex and do you have opinions like that or different?
- If you are lonely, what have you thought about doing to manage that and what have you tried? How has it worked?
- If you are missing the touching and intimacy of earlier years, have you found ways to bring touch back to your life?

TIPS FOR EIGHTYSOMETHINGS

- Remember we are sexual beings and it is normal to be interested in sex throughout life.
- For those of you who are part of a couple, remember sex in the eighties is all about intimacy and there are many ways to be intimate beyond intercourse.
- Talk to your partner about your needs and wants even if it takes some courage to bring it up. If you yearn for more affection, tell your partner.
- If you are missing touch, consider massages, visiting with grandchildren, and neighboring pets.

TIPS FOR FAMILIES

- Talk to your eightysomething about loneliness. Share something about times you have been lonely in your life and talk about your coping mechanisms.

- Ask your eightysomething parent or relative who is now a widow or widower if they would like to talk for a while about their spouse. Looking at photographs is an easy way to begin and can bring sheer joy.
- If they are in a new relationship, your support can mean a lot. Or if you have concerns about the relationship, express them frankly.

CHAPTER 7

GRANDPARENTING

Grandchildren have been called the romance of old age. And while it is true that grandparenting is usually one the most delightful and meaningful experiences of life, when you are an eightysomething, it is different from when you were younger. Not only are they enchanting and adorable, they are our legacy. But they can also break your heart. The number of children living with grandparents has doubled since 1970.[1]

Jane, eighty-two, is one of those eightysomething grandparents in the United States who has grandchildren living with her. Sometimes a grandparent moves in with adult children, and sometimes, as in Jane's case, the adult children and grandchildren move in with elderly parents. Her household consists of herself; her husband; her daughter, Ellen; Ellen's husband, Wesley; and their two children, Phoebe, six, and Tobias, three. Wesley has a job in a city a thousand miles away and comes home every other weekend. "It may be hard to believe, but we are really enjoying it," Jane told me.

Jane and her husband live in a large green Victorian house perched on a shady hill in a suburb of New York. On the day in June when I visited, the grass had not been mowed and shrubs were so overgrown as to practically conceal the house. Jane met me at the kitchen door and led me to the living room, passing six or seven large cardboard boxes overflowing with LEGOs, wooden blocks, Lincoln logs, dolls, doll houses, and stuffed animals. I disrupted a fat black and orange cat to sit down on a faded velvet chair.

Jane is a ruddy woman with a hearty laugh who radiates well-being. She explained that Ellen and her family moved in "temporarily" five years ago, while Wesley looked for a new job. But since his job situation remains uncertain, it has never been a good time for them to move out. Jane said it works well since Ellen does the lion's share of caring for the kids and she also buys the groceries and cooks dinners. Jane provides childcare when Ellen goes out.

Jane explained that she spends lots of time with the kids and she loves it. She reads books to them and they sing songs. The kids have no computer tablets and there is no TV in the house. The kids put on puppet shows, dress up in costumes from an enormous chest out in the hall, and stage fights with fake swords. Phoebe, the six-year-old, has an inquisitive mind, so Jane and she have lots of conversations about such things as why trees can stand up and not fall down, and whether there is life in other parts of the universe or not.

This rapturous picture of family life seemed too good to be true, so I asked Jane about the down sides of having the grandkids live with them. After a moment of thinking, Jane said, "Well, it is messy." She went on to say that spending so much time with kids means she doesn't have much time for herself. Also, the kids get up very early, at around six o'clock, and are noisy. Mostly, she only wishes she could do more for Ellen, who has even less time for herself than she has. They have never talked about rent or when Ellen and her family will move out.

Jane had no serious complaints. It seemed to be working. I worried, though, that she has not set any boundaries on the living arrangements and wondered if she isn't doing more that she really wants to do.

My visit with Jane was like time-travel, back to the early twentieth century to the pre-digital world of books and music, caring adults, and plenty of time for the grandkids. It made me nostalgic for my own childhood. But, of course, that world doesn't exist for the vast majority of children in the United States today. I wondered, too, how Jane's grandkids will fit in at school. Will their lack of screen experience make it hard for them to connect to their classmates? And at the same time, I wish that every grandparent could provide their grandchildren with even just a touch of the old-fashioned magic that Jane was providing.

Thanksgiving at my grandmother's house was happy, too, as I remember it. The house smelled of roasting turkey and apple pie. The grownups talked loudly and cheerfully about the past. I have clung to that image of a happy, multigenerational family all my life. Similar images are powerful for most people, as well. No matter how different the reality of their family might be, they continue to yearn for that dream.

But what is grandparenting really like for eightysomethings today? Never in all of history have so many people lived into their eighties. In the past, children usually grew up knowing only one or two of their own grandparents. The others had died. But they usually knew the ones still alive well because they lived close by. Today's children may have three or four living grandparents and even one or two great-grandparents, but some of them typically live far away. This is due to the far greater mobility today compared to the past.

The role of grandparents is more important today than ever. With smaller families today, children have fewer siblings, fewer cousins, and fewer aunts and uncles. Their only link to an older generation may be grandparents.

Another change from the past is how unusual it is for grandchildren and grandparents to be living in the same household, as in Jane's case. Actually, the numbers have gone up slightly in recent years as grandparents have needed to step in to help after a divorce because of the rising cost of housing, or the drug addiction of a parent.[2]

Grandparenting for those in their eighties is not as it was in their seventies. Their circumstances and capabilities have changed. For example, when I came to live in the retirement community I stopped hosting my family for Thanksgiving. And I have done almost no childcare these last four years since there are no little ones. Today my grandkids range from ages eleven to twenty-eight, and as my grandkids grow older, there are possibilities for new kinds of satisfying relationships.

The stories of Margie, Clark, Marshall, and Audrey illustrate some of the different kinds of experiences that eightysomething grandparents report.

Margie's experiences with her grandchildren over the last twenty years included a number of disappointments as well as many happy times. Barely five feet tall, Margie walks with a limp but also with an expression of determination. She and her husband live in Providence, Rhode Island, as does one of her two sons and his wife and their two children, Tate, twenty, and May, seventeen. May is autistic. While May has some ability to talk, she can only respond to a few simple questions that are familiar to her. She has frequent meltdowns and is difficult to manage outside of her home.

Margie, eighty-three, has tried to be helpful with May, but her son and daughter-in-law preferred to deal with May alone. "They have never trusted us with May," she said. "Now that we are older grandparents and since my stroke four years ago, I am not agile, I can understand their reluctance to let us care for her. Mostly, I am just sorry about how their whole family's lives have been narrowed—no trips, little social life. I also worry about what will happen to May when she ages out of school." Tate, May's older brother, adores her, but Margie reports he has never brought any friends to the house. Margie catches a rare glimpse of him now and then when he is home from college.

Margie talks with her other grandson who is thirteen and lives in Chicago on Skype every Sunday night and she looks forward to his family's visits three or four times a year.

Margie laments her lack of day-to-day contact with all the grandchildren. Of course, things have been complicated with May's autism and now with her own stoke. But still, she can't help feeling a bit rejected.

Clark, eighty-three, a former lumberjack who lives in a trailer near Yellowstone National Park in Montana, is even more unconnected to his grandchildren than Margie. Until two years ago he was cutting down trees but now he is working at a sawmill. He told me he is unusual because he married and divorced the same woman twice. He has nine grandchildren; six of them live in Florida and two live in Idaho. He never sees the Florida grandchildren and rarely sees the two who live in Idaho. He does see one grandson who also works at the sawmill, but Clark doesn't often talk with him. "Not as much as I'd like anyway," he added.

This kind of distance between grandparents and grandkids is common today. Studies report that only one in five grandchildren spend much time with their grandparents.[3] Several grandparents told me that when their grandkids do turn up, they are often looking for money. Most grandchildren, it seems, are not curious about their grandparents' lives. Many don't even know the names of all their grandparents. However, there is also some research showing that grandchildren almost always experience their grandparents as loving and caring.

Grandchildren can also bring pain and conflict as well as great joy to a family, as Marshall's story of his grandchildren illustrates. Marshall, eighty-four, lives in a small city in New Hampshire close to his two kids, four of his five grandchildren, and three great-grandchildren. His wife died the year before I interviewed him, but his kids continue to visit him on Sunday afternoons. They hang out on his deck talking, while the great-grandkids play in the yard. Their visits are the highlight of Marshall's week.

It hasn't always been so easy because one grandchild, Samantha, has had problems with drugs and addiction for decades. Marshall explained that Samantha did some terrible things to her mother, Marshall's daughter, Candace. She used to steal money from her for drugs, curse at her, and even spit in her face. Candace had to call the police on several occasions. Candace, accompanied by Marshall, took Samantha to court a few years ago and Samantha spent some time in jail. Marshall says what Samantha did to her mother was unforgiveable, and to this day he won't have anything to do with her. But he is grateful for all the other grand-children who are so loving and close.

Audrey, eighty-four, is another grandparent, like Clark, who lives far away from her grandchildren, although she has always found ways to stay connected to them. Besides holidays and birthdays, every summer, the entire family, in later years consisting of her two children and their spouses and five grandchildren, spent time together at a cottage in Maine. They have years and years of wonderful memories and photos to document it all. But now the grandkids have jobs, Audrey's husband is dead, and Maine has not happened the last two years.

Audrey also took each of her three granddaughters on a trip when they were fifteen. The last trip, when Audrey was eighty-two, was less of a success. Her granddaughter Madison came down with a nasty cold and wasn't interested in seeing the sights of San Francisco. Even after a trip to a doctor and some antibiotics, she just wanted to stay in the hotel room and watch TV. They cut the trip short by a day. Audrey remembers a man at the airport looking at the two of them, and saying to Madison, "What are you doing with that old lady?" And Audrey was wondering the same thing. She realized she herself no longer had the stamina to deal with a sick and sullen teenager. When Audrey told me about this comment, I thought about how rude, how hurtful, and how ageist that man was.

Audrey has held onto her old ways of doing things. And as an eighty-something, grandparenting, like everything else, needs to be adapted to current capabilities. But what made me feel sad about her as we talked was how she bought into that man's comment that a young teenager wouldn't want to be with her, an old lady.

Another part of the story is about those who have no grandchildren, like Julianne who is eighty-one. I wondered what that was like for her.

Julianne, whose husband died a year ago, tells me that one of her two daughters never got married and the other one never wanted any children. The married one who is now fifty-six lives in Alaska. Julianne said it was many years before she knew for sure there would be no grandchildren and gave up hope.

When I ask how she feels about not having grandchildren now, she said she is so used to it and it happened so slowly that it isn't painful most of the time. What does hurt is that at Christmas she just doesn't have that much family. It feels empty with just her and her single daughter. She said it also feels bad when she meets new people because usually the second or third question they ask her is, "How many grandchildren do you have?" And if she says, "None" there is a painful silence. So she has learned to say, cheerfully, "None, but I do have a grand dog." And they all laugh and that works for everybody.

Julianne is typical of the many eightysomethings without grandchildren when she reports that it doesn't hurt on a day-to-day basis. We humans adjust to whatever our conditions actually are. But she admitted, "I do realize every now and then that I have missed out on one of life's most important joys."

I, like most who are grandparents, am profoundly grateful for my ten grandchildren and for the richness that they have brought into my life. It was sheer bliss holding my one-day-old grandbabies one after another. And all the wonderful times that followed—but that was in the past.

In my eighties, as far as the grandchildren are concerned, it has been more talking and less doing. I couldn't play soccer any more with Asher, and besides, at eleven, he didn't really want to play with his grandmother, either. Today I can't even give him a run for his money in ping-pong. But as the grandchildren become young adults setting out into the world on their own, I have had all sorts of ways to connect to them.

Most recently, my phone conversations with Jonathan have been special. A recent college graduate, he is spending two years in Hong Kong teaching English at a university. We have talked a number of times for over an hour. He has told me about the ten-year-old girl he is tutoring, about his classes, about his travels to mainland China and Vietnam, his girlfriend, and the Chinese professor he is working for. He has, in short, opened a window into his life and let me in. What a privilege. With today's social media bringing endless possibilities to communicate, distance isn't the same obstacle to having a close relationship as it was in the past.

Grandparents play many roles in the lives of their grandchildren even as they age. They are caregivers, trip leaders, confidantes, advocates, providers of financial assistance, replacements for a missing parent, providers of a place to gather, and family anchors. There are dozens of other possible roles, too.

Sometimes, what limits eightysomething grandparents' relationships is not distance or their declining health but the stereotypes of old people they have accepted. Audrey feels old and assumes her granddaughter might not enjoy her company. The media doesn't help as grandparents are often depicted as childish, silly, sexless, and powerless. They are expected to be always cheerful, undemanding, and caring. Worse still, they are often invisible. Can you think of a film that revolves around a grandchild and a grandparent? *Heidi* is all that comes to my mind. Violet, the grandmother that Maggie Smith played in *Downton Abbey,* provided a welcome counter example of a forceful, loving, and witty grandmother. I think many grandparents lack the imagination to see the important roles they could play in their grandkids' lives.

In today's world, grandparents often have more investment in their relationship with their grandchildren than the grandchildren have in them. The relations are often not symmetrical. This is natural, because it can be said that love runs downhill. Parents adore their children with a love unlike any other. And grandparents adore their grandchildren. They have more at stake, more to gain it may seem, from a close relationship, while the grandchildren are trying to grow up and be independent.

Some grandchildren turn to their grandparents for support throughout their lives and, especially, when they are in conflict with their parents as they try to separate from them. They often find warm acceptance and nurturance that the parents may not be able to provide.

Grandparents often have great investment in their grandchildren whether they are close by or far away. They are their insurance of some kind of continuity after they are dead; they are their tie with the future. In most cases, they carry their DNA. They provide emotional fulfillment to them; they are young people given to them to love. They provide a peek into the wonderful world of the young.

Grandchildren also provide a second chance. Often grandparents look back and see that as parents they were terribly stressed much of the time, too often impatient and preoccupied. Or, maybe even absent from the scene. But by the time they are eighty, almost everyone has lots of time and is moving slowly. They are patient. They savor the opportunity to spend time with their grandchildren. They can be more caring and affirming than they were with their children. And even if they rarely see any of their grandchildren, the lives of eightysomethings are enhanced just by the fact that they exist. And when they are together, grandparents are now able to be truly present, to actually experience the joy of being there with a grandchild.

CONVERSATION STARTERS
- What kind of relationship do you have with each of your grandchildren?
- How has grandparenting changed for you now that you are in your eighties?

- How do you keep in touch with your grandchildren? Do you reach out to them?
- Can you think about times in recent years when you felt particularly close to a grandchild?

TIPS FOR FAMILIES

- If you are part of a multigenerational household, be sure you have created guidelines for how things are done and what are the rules of the house. This is important for joint vacations together, too.
- Make an effort to include eightysomethings in family events like recitals, birthdays, and graduations.
- Encourage your eightysomething parent to stay in touch with all the grandchildren, perhaps inviting them to visit one at a time.
- Help your eightysomething learn how to use social media and how to text so it will be easier for them to stay in touch. Help them when their technology isn't working.

CHAPTER 8

CAREGIVERS

There are forty million people in the United States today, mostly unpaid, taking care of others, mostly their relatives. They provide $470 billion in services.[1] When a family member falls ill, they step up and become a caretaker. They find themselves performing tasks they never imagined they would ever be doing: giving shots, changing catheters, and dressing wounds. They learn on the job. Some of these caregivers are people in their eighties who are caring for a spouse, a child, or a sibling. Caregiving is always difficult, but the challenges it presents for caretakers who are in their eighties are even more daunting.

This chapter focuses on what the experience of caretaking is like for eightysomethings. The References section at the end of the book provides references with medical and financial information that caretakers may need. This chapter is focused on the emotional ups and downs that are embedded in the caregiving process and how to navigate them successfully. What makes caretaking go well and what are pitfalls to avoid?

Connie's story is a good place to begin. Connie's husband died four months before I interviewed her at the retirement community where she now lives. Connie, eighty-seven, took care of Bart, her husband, for ten years as he slowly succumbed to the ravages of Parkinson's disease. The day I spoke with her she was sitting in her pajamas and a bathrobe relaxing in a recliner. She is a warm, grandmotherly woman with curly white hair and a smile that rarely leaves her face. She began by telling me that she and Bart had been crazy about each other: "We did almost everything together."

"It all started when Bart just couldn't control his shaking hands and the coffee would slurp out," she said. Finally, after some months, when a neurologist told them it was Parkinson's, Bart's reaction was to tell Connie, "I couldn't answer the doctor's questions. I felt stupid."

Bart's shame didn't go away. He didn't want anyone to know about his diagnosis, including his four kids. He stopped going to his men's group and to church. He couldn't stand anyone feeling sorry for him and just wanted to stay at home.

This kind of shame in response to an illness is not uncommon, especially with men who are used to being in control and who are not used to talking about their vulnerabilities. Yet withdrawing from friends and family makes it more difficult for everyone.

Connie was determined to take care of Bart and to do it all by herself. "I can do this," she said to herself. Two years later, Bart still didn't want anyone else in the house to help out, although he needed constant help. Connie was providing it all. She was helping Bart dress, helping him with his medicines, and helping him get to the bathroom several times each night. "I was tired but I still thought I could manage. I would tell everyone, 'Don't worry about me.'"

One day one of his doctors asked her how she was doing, and she burst into tears. "He told me I must get help. It took the doctor telling me to get help to be able to do it."

A few years later, Bart and Connie had a small army of helpers. They had six caregivers from a local agency that came in shifts most of the day and night. Besides that, there was a network of professional care that included Bart's doctor, the neurologist, an urologist, a physical therapist, an occupational therapist, and a dermatologist. When Bart took a serious fall, a surgeon was added to the list. That's not counting the four children who helped from time to time. Connie said, "These people were literally lifesavers—his life and mine. I remain profoundly grateful."

Connie went on to say life was not all sad and dreary. "Each morning Bart would greet me with a long hug. By then we were not in the same bedroom. Several of the caregivers told me they were jealous of how much we seemed to love each other."

Connie went on, "A lot did change for us as I had to take over so much. There was scheduling all the appointments and getting Bart to and from, organizing the shifts of the caregivers, keeping the children up to date, taking trips to the emergency room, managing the family finances which I had never done before, along with the house maintenance, insurance and taxes, all new to me."

Caretaking produces dramatic and subtle changes in a couple's relationship as you can see from Connie and Bart's story. Before his illness, Bart saw himself as the head of the family whose role was provide for them and take care of them. After his illness, he had to learn how to let people care for him. Connie, who had always let Bart run the show, had to learn how to be more assertive and take on more executive functions. Bart had to learn how to be a good *patient* and Connie had to get comfortable being a *manager*.

By the time Bart died, Connie felt like she had become a different person. While she misses him all the time, today she enjoys staying in bed half the morning knowing there is nothing she has to do.

Flynn, eighty-five, is another devoted caretaker. He lives in a retirement village. "I look at it as payback time," explained Flynn to me as we discussed what it is like for him to be the caregiver of his wife, Dede. "During our marriage we always moved wherever my job took us from east to west several times. I feel bad because I had always said she could choose where we lived in retirement. And now Dede is in a wheelchair and has lost the ability to speak in the last year." Flynn has been caring for her for seven years since she fell and experienced significant brain damage. "I am planning on keeping her here in the cottage no matter what," he said.

Flynn explained that he thinks he was born to be a caretaker, "It is in my genes. It is my purpose in life and I enjoy taking care of Dede. We have always been good friends. Even now when she doesn't speak, she still has a good sense of humor and she is good company. I want her to have some social life so I invite people over for a glass of wine a couple of times a week." I saw how completely Flynn identified with Dede's well-being.

When I asked Flynn what has been the hardest part of being a caretaker, he responded that, "I feel so sad that Dede is not able to speak up and complain. I worry most about what will happen to her, if something should happen to me. I had a mild stroke that was not too serious, but it scared me. I can't do emails any more. After the stroke my doctor told me I needed to get help to relieve some of my stress. So now the aides dress and feed Dede. I've begun going away once a month."

Although Flynn, like Connie, had no training or preparation for the job of caregiver, for him, it seemed easy, natural. But he, too, had to learn the hard way that a lopsided lifestyle of self-sacrifice was just not sustainable. He still doesn't fully understand that self-care is part of being an effective caretaker. And I am not sure he understands what self-care means and how it might improve his life.

Not all people have the resources like Connie and Flynn to hire aides to help them out as their spouse needs more care than they can provide. Medicare and Medicaid do provide help and care, and there are community resources like Visiting Nurses and Meals on Wheels. But many caregivers have to keep on going even when their own health is compromised.

A shift in roles also happened with Melissa and Lex, a couple who are both eighty-one. Lex, a social worker who had worked at a nonprofit agency, was diagnosed with a rare form of cancer of the blood three years ago. Melissa began our interview by telling me, "I am the luckiest person in the world because I am taking care of Lex, and he is such a special person. I am not sure how long I will have him but for now we are still such partners. I still want to know what he thinks about things."

Now caretaking takes up most of Melissa's time. She has given up her other activities to be with Lex twenty-four/seven except for an hour and a half each week when their daughter comes to the house to give her a break. "Our routines take a lot of time," she said. "In the morning I help Lex dress—getting his shoes on is especially difficult—and I make sure he takes his meds. This routine takes a couple of hours, and the bedtime routine is about the same." At this point she takes a detour and tells me about a catalog, oddly called Gold Violin, where you can get all the supplies you need to take care of someone with problems of incontinence and thousands of other kinds of equipment you never knew existed or thought you would need.

Melissa continued, "Things changed over time. I now manage the finances; that is new for me since I am slowing down, too. Things really changed, though, when I had to go to the hospital with pneumonia. While I was in the hospital, Lex fell sometime during the night and couldn't get up. It wasn't until the next day that one of the kids arrived and found him. I now keep both kids up to date on the situation as it changes."

Then Lex began resisting taking his meds:

> I would try to get him to take them and he didn't like being told what to do. I tried to hide my annoyance but Lex picked up on it. We began having little fights over silly things all the time. He said he didn't like Bossy Melissa. He had taught me that "dependency can breed hostility," explaining that we adults like to be in control and that being a patient is frustrating. And now here we were acting it out. I realized I needed to be kind and loving all the time, but it is hard. I try to be cheerful, or what passes for cheerful, but often I just don't have the energy. Most of the time, I should add, he is in good spirits and takes all his meds.

I have learned to let a lot of things go. I realize it doesn't matter if we are late for most places. I find it is okay with me to not have time outside the house, but I miss time for my own reading. If we had more money, we could have more caretakers to help him with showers and to give me a break to get out of the house. But it's okay.

The annoyance and frustrations that both Lex and Melissa feel are part of every long-term caretaking relationship. Our society still glorifies independence and makes many people feel if they are dependent, they are failures. Ideally, a couple takes turns being the one who is dependent and the one giving care. But when there is a serious illness and long-term dependence, it is no longer possible to maintain balance. However, if caretakers are aware of the dynamics of dependency, neither patient nor caretaker will be so unsettled when they feel frustrated and angry with their beloved partner.

For me, another difficult part of my experience taking care of John was trying to find my way through the maze that is the healthcare system today. It was a struggle to get the right care for John.

After he had been on dialysis for a year, John had a small stroke , sadly on his eighty-seventh birthday. At the local hospital they thought at first that he had had a heart attack which meant he needed to go to a different hospital. Once there, a few tests showed that his heart was not involved and that his issue was a stroke. But it turned out there was no bed in the stroke unit, so he was kept at the heart unit. I was told that once a day, a doctor from the stroke unit would check on him. On several days I waited all day and no doctor came. Maybe they came at midnight. I didn't know what to do except to keep asking about the doctor.

A week later, when it came time for John to leave the hospital, the discharge person wanted him to go to a place thirty-five miles from our home. What seemed important to me was to get him placed near me at the nursing home attached to our retirement community where we would be close together. That was what he wanted. But the discharge worker was adamant that the place she was suggesting was where he should go. I felt helplessly lost again in the bureaucracy even though I was a social worker and should know how to push the system. I saw she didn't understand our priorities or values. She would simply proceed with her plan.

That night I called my son, Dan, and said I really needed him to come and help me get his dad out of this place and somewhere close to home. He arrived the next morning and we spent the day calling to find a skilled nursing facility nearby. At about noon, a bed in the skilled nursing facility where I hoped he could go, the one attached to our retirement community, became available for him. At that point we learned that we needed four different people to sign off in order to spring him loose that day. We started making calls. And more calls. Finally, at five that afternoon, we got the last sign off, and by nightfall he was in a bed at the nursing home that is part of our retirement community.

There was one final bit of nightmare to that day. As I was driving home a few minutes behind John who was in an ambulance, I saw his ambulance and another car pulled off to the side of the road. My heart skipped a beat. What had happened? It turned out the car had rear ended the ambulance, but no one was hurt.

This experience is how I learned once again that, yes, you do have to advocate for your loved one who is ill, and it is difficult to do. I relearned, too, how important it is to understand that most of the difficulties encountered are system problems, not problems caused by mean or uncaring individuals. The system is often rigid and bureaucratic.

The squeaky wheel gets the grease. You will also need to call on your friends and families. In my case, a friend of my son Ben is a kidney specialist. He came and talked with me several times while providing information about what I should expect. He made it easier for me to have the strength to carry on.

Caregiving is not all difficulties. Those who are caregivers know how important what they are doing is. Caring for a loved one provides purpose and meaning. The caregiver is usually too busy to get depressed. They have work to do. Caretakers learn about self-care, how to ask for help, and how to be an advocate. They become more patient, flexible, and empathic.

Caretakers are truly the unsung heroes of our time.

CONVERSATION STARTERS

- Have you been a caretaker? What has it been like for you?
- How about your experience as a patient? How did that change you?
- What do you do now for self-care, whether you are currently sick or well, caretaking or cared for?
- In what ways did you grow and change from being a caretaker or a patient?

TIPS FOR FAMILIES

- Talk to your eightysomething about the status of their health, ask about what help they have and what more they may need.
- Keep talking about self-care, why it matters, and what it is.
- When your eightysomething gets angry or irritated, remember it is hard to be dependent and being eighty usually means you are becoming more dependent.
- Check on whether they need some help in navigating the maze that is our healthcare system today. Where are they stymied? Are they avoiding taking care of a situation that needs attention? Help them figure out what to do.

CHAPTER 9

A SHRINKING WORLD

One way of looking at the entire process of aging is to see it as a journey toward a smaller world. Helen Lake, the author of the book *Old Age*, calls it a journey into simplicity. This idea of moving toward a simpler, smaller world catches many aspects of the eightysomething experience. Their bodies shrink, they move to smaller homes, travel less, give away more, and simplify their lifestyles. But there are vast differences among eightysomethings themselves regarding their attitude toward this journey; some of them embrace it and others resist it vigorously.

I'll begin with height. Most people have lost an inch or two of their height by the time they turn eighty. Some lose more. Take me, for example. As a young woman, I used to feel tall when I measured five feet six and three quarters inches. Today, I am only five foot three. When someone the other day referred to me as a "small person" I did a double take. Me? Surely not? This is an aspect of my aging that I don't like, but it is one of the changes that is not worth complaining about.

Downsizing, on the other hand, is a major change. Many eightysomethings move to a smaller place, move in with a child, or go to a retirement community, an assisted living facility, or a nursing home. But even more of them stay put in their homes and resist any move. Most people want to age in place, to stay in their own home if they possibly can. According to the US Census Bureau, only slightly more than 5 percent of elders live in nursing homes despite the common impression that the number is much larger.[1]

Both financial capability and health issues are critical factors in determining whether and where eightysomethings move. Retirement communities can be very pricey and are often not an option. Nursing homes are viewed as the last resort and resisted by most people. What this means is that some eightysomethings stay in their homes far longer than it is reasonable or safe for them to do.

The village movement for seniors provides new options for people who want to stay in their home. It has spawned innovative grassroots organizations which provide the necessary support services to seniors wishing to remain at home. Beacon Hill Village, in Boston, founded in 2002, was the first of these village organizations. For a modest annual fee of less than a thousand dollars, a village organization will provide information and access to local home maintenance resources, learning options, and social events—many of the same services that are offered in residential retirement communities. In 2017, there were over 350 villages around the country that were already active or were in development.[2]

Eightysomethings not only downsize their homes, but for most of them, the geographical space they move about in also begins to get smaller. They travel less and spend far more time at home than ever before. After John and I moved to the retirement community, we rarely went to the movies anymore or out to eat. Walking was so hard for John. Driving in the car was uncomfortable for him, too, so we made many fewer visits to our kids who were scattered up and down the east coast. It was just more relaxing for us to stay put. Many eightysomethings find sleeping in new places is complicated because of their fixed bedtime routines and health issues.

In terms of friends, the world of eightysomethings is vastly smaller than in previous decades. People treasure their longtime friends but half the people in their age group have died. Some people in their eighties become very set in their ways and don't want to meet any new people, while others go ahead and make new friends, often because they have moved to a new location. This can be a happy surprise.

Almost every eightysomething has made the transition from seeking to acquire more stuff to wanting to get rid of some of their possessions. I think this is because taking care of things becomes burdensome and also there is a growing pleasure in simplicity that seems to be part of the aging process for most people. But actually following through on their intentions is another story. Resistance to the actual process of letting go of possessions can be fierce.

Rachel, eighty-four, is one who avoids the journey to a smaller living space and is also resistant to giving up any of her stuff. She and her husband of more than sixty years have lived in a house in the suburbs of New York and another house on Cape Cod. She tells me that essentially she hasn't changed anything in either of the houses in fifty years. "It is a lot of work, too much." she added in a slightly whiney voice. "Time is closing in on me and it weighs on me. I am not organized and not letting go of anything. I am anxious about this all the time and am just waiting for something disastrous to happen."

Rachel tells me that, while she enjoys being active on several boards and professional groups related to her former career as an urban planner, she despises her exercise class. She only takes it in order to stay healthy, so she won't have to change her life in any way.

Edith, like Rachel, has been unsuccessful in her attempts to pare down her possessions. She is the busy woman whom you met in chapter 4, who is a member of four book groups. When her husband became ill, they moved into a nearby retirement community. But Edith could not face putting the house on the market—so she didn't. While her husband was alive she made trips back to the house each day for a few hours. But after he died, she found she wanted to spend most of her days not at the retirement community but at her old house. She hosts her book groups there and has friends over for lunch at the house. She loves to cook at the house and still has a garden. She told me, "I am hoping I can swing both places for a while. I just can't seem to move ahead and put the house on the market or settle into the retirement community. Luckily, I am not a worrier."

I, too, dreaded for months having to give away most of my things when we moved from our house to the retirement community. And to this day I feel nostalgic about that house on Independence Road nestled among tall pine trees and overgrown rhododendrons. But how I actually felt giving away many of my possessions was a total surprise when I actually did it.

As we prepared to move, we invited our four sons, their wives, and the grandchildren to come to the house and select whatever they would like from the stuff we had accumulated over fifty years. We put green stickers on everything we were taking ourselves and the rest was up for grabs. We gave each of the kids and grandkids their own color stickers to put on the things they wanted. If several people wanted the same object, we asked them to work it out.

The day took on the feel of a party or grand scavenger hunt with people buzzing around the house. I noticed that Julie, my granddaughter who was in the military, surprisingly wanted a set of flowery salad plates, and Sarah took all the beat-up pots and pans. Unbelievable. No one wanted the tea set. Oh, well. But all my mother's watercolors were all selected. It was a roller coaster of emotions—joy, laughter, sadness. They were all on their best behavior, avoiding bickering and conflict. That in itself made the giving away so much easier and so much fun.

What was also unexpected—it was shocking, actually—was that after we moved I never gave another thought to all those possessions I had given away. It was out of sight, out of mind. It felt okay to have fewer things. Actually, I felt lighter and freer without all those things. I will admit that I did miss quite a few of the books that I didn't bring.

This pleasure I feel in having less, I learned, is typical of most eighty-somethings. It really is true that "less is more." In your eighties, anyway. I believe this because as we age and our death approaches, we begin to prepare for our death in many ways. Getting rid of stuff is one of these ways Helen Lake says we all have a choice of pathways as we age. One path is a continuation, a repetition of the way we have lived our life; the other is a new way of being, a turning away from the accustomed efforts toward a new, significant journey inward. Old age can be a time when one can be "free of instructions, ambition and the pose of wisdom." For those who choose to let go, to embrace the gifts reserved for old age, "old age becomes freedom, becomes a dance, becomes the laughter that lies on the other side of letting go."[3]

Bernice, eighty-eight, is one who has been quite successful at choosing a new way of being that works for her in her eighties. Before retiring, Bernice was a professor of history and had collected a number of oral histories in Appalachia. She told me, "My life changed in almost every way in my eighties. I am a strong person, but now I am always really tired, without energy. I always thought I should do more, but I have found out that determination didn't always work."

Bernice recognized she had to change. She sold her house that none of the children wanted or could afford and moved to an apartment. She gave most of her furniture and china to her daughters and found to her surprise that seeing it in their houses gave her enormous pleasure. When she realized she was moving too slowly getting rid of her papers and belongings, she hired one of her daughters to help with the job. She said, "I have been able to change, especially important has been getting over that nagging feeling that I should always be doing more. When I clean out a single drawer, I feel proud. I know it is an accomplishment."

Now Bernice is also far more selective when deciding how to spend her time. She is careful not to schedule too much, eliminating all but the most meaningful activities. Although most of her good friends have died, she has been able to make a few new friends. But, she said, "I am careful just to see people I like very much. And I am different now because I don't talk politics anymore and I avoid being confrontational. I stay in touch with the grandchildren and others, but I no longer think I have wonderful advice for them all."

Bernice is clearly trimming her life to focus on essentials, and she has become realistic about what is possible for her. She has stopped giving instructions and relinquished the belief that she has all the answers. In Helen Luke's language, she has given up the pose of wisdom and she is clearly taking control of her journey.

Helen Luke's view of old age, as bringing new possibilities, resonates with my own optimistic worldview. The journey inward, however, is not the only possibility or choice as we age. It is also not the path for all people. But I am clear that holding onto old patterns can't work forever. Rachel is already quite anxious and apprehensive about the future. Edith is happy but knows at some level she is being foolhardy to keep both houses. When I spoke with them, neither of them saw any appeal in change or going in a new direction. Change to them means loss, only loss. I hope they can learn to let go.

The idea that we keep developing, even in our last stages of life, is fairly new. Until recently it was assumed that life after sixty was just the loss of brain cells and brain power year by year. Most experts today believe that as we age we have the potential to grow and develop in ways that were not imagined in the past. Thomas Moore, a former monk and author of many spiritual books, adds to the picture of development as we age, describing it as ongoing alchemy. He suggests it makes sense to allow the fool in each of us to step forward, so we can see beyond what is obvious and get to mysteries that appear when life is less focused and controlled.

Agnes Rose, eighty-eight, a nun who lives in Ohio, has travelled far along the pathway not only toward simplicity but also toward inner spiritual development. She said, "When I first came to the retirement home,

I, as usual, volunteered to do what was needed. I worked in the office on the finances, cleaned up the craft room, and ran groups for the sisters where they could just sit and talk about their lives."

Agnes Rose continued,

> I used to be extroverted, wanting to make everything right. I used to think the best thing I could do was bring to people my laughter, my sense of humor. When I told a story and they all laughed, that was an ultimate pleasure. Now I am shifting to being more of an introvert. I have no need to achieve. I am more interior now. I don't miss being so involved and I don't mind being alone in my room for long periods of time. I feel a certain serenity that is new.
>
> In terms of my belongings, I have narrowed, narrowed. Anything I own is in this room. As a young nun, I used to travel with a single trunk, but then I would accumulate things wherever I went. I don't want to have a bunch of stuff around when I die, so I have given most of my things to my nephews. It feels wonderful to have so little.

Some of the sisters at the retirement home, she explained, are very sick and others have dementia: "Death walks gently among us. Some sisters are like ancient parchment—so fragile, but we know how to handle them. What really matters, I believe, is to be there for others, to be present in their sorrows."

She added, "What I still have kept is a little clay figure of a monk with an empty bowl. He is my symbol of becoming emptied out. I don't have plans anymore and I don't give advice anymore. I used to pontificate. I feel I am being gently transformed into myself."

Agnes Rose has arrived at simplicity. She is enjoying now the freedom and the dance that follow in the wake of letting go. I thought to myself that kind of freedom is not easily attained. Many of us eightysomethings cling ever more tightly to our old patterns. I doubt I will ever be an inward person. Here I am, trying hard to finish this book, still wrapped up in getting things done, holding on to activities and buying even more books. That may be who I really am. But I admit the image of the Agnes Rose's clay monk holding an empty bowl beckons me on. It has an allure. "But not yet," I say, "not yet."

CONVERSATION STARTERS

- In terms of possessions, where are you in process of wanting to get rid of some of your things and, also, in actually doing it?
- How has your world become smaller in terms of geography and friends? And what has that been like for you?
- Do you see yourself on a journey toward simplicity? In what aspects of your life? Are you becoming more spiritual?
- Which material object that you have means most to you and why?

TIPS FOR FAMILIES

- Getting rid of possessions can be an overwhelming process for most eightysomethings. This is a time for families to offer to help out. It will make an enormous difference.
- If your eightysomething is making unwise choices about where they live or their possessions, remember they have the right to make poor choices.
- Have your eightysomething take you around their home and explain which objects mean most to them and what is the story behind each of them. It will be fun for both of you.
- Explore with them what they are moving toward.

CHAPTER 10

PAST, FUTURE, AND PRESENT

We are sipping mimosas and our plates are piled with food. It is the New Year's Day buffet brunch at my retirement community. Eight of us are gathered: six eightysomethings and two people in their seventies. The conversation begins with the weather. It is a frigid eight degrees and will stay that way for several days. Lots to complain about there. Someone comments randomly, "You can never have too much bacon."

One man is wearing some new-fangled hearing aids that look like ear-muffs. Another man, who also has hearing loss, wants to learn more about them. He says, "But that is probably too nurdly a topic for us to discuss in detail at this social occasion." We all laugh at the word nurdly.

This takes us to engineers and a joke from the guy with the fancy hearing aids. "Optimists say the glass is half full, pessimists say it is half empty, and engineers says the glass is too small." We all laugh again.

We make a few toasts and then someone asks, "Who here is making New Year's resolutions?" A large woman says she is starting a diet the next day.

This was a typical eightysomething conversation—sticking closely to the here and now. It is interesting what was omitted. There were few complaints about health despite many aches and pains. Nothing about the long years *before* coming to the retirement facility. Nothing about all the missing spouses, three of whom have died recently. That day, as the year begins, during that time of looking before and after, these eightysomethings said nothing about the past or the future . . . except for the upcoming diet.

Eightysomethings, indeed, have a very long past to think about. However, many find themselves quite alone with their memories. Wherever they live, at their home of many years, at a new home, or in a retirement community, they live with neighbors with whom they may have no shared past. Few people around them knew them as a younger person. Eightysomethings have lost at least half, if not more, of their friends. Like those of us at the New Year's buffet, many eightysomethings are without their spouses. Even their children only remember some of the years of their long lives.

Eightysomethings also often have a surprising lack of knowledge about the past life of the people they are spending time with currently. Take Bob, for example, a man my husband and I had dinner with at least eight or nine times at our retirement community. Bob's hearing was seriously impaired, so we needed to practically shout for him to hear us. And when he spoke, half the time I didn't know what he had said because of his heavy accent. Usually it was about the food and the wait staff. So when he died, I was flabbergasted to read his obituary that took up three whole columns in the *New York Times*. Bob was a world-famous-engineer who had played a key role in the development of the computer and artificial intelligence in the 1950s. I'd had no idea.

Why didn't I know more about him? Because the past doesn't mean that much at a retirement community. Whether you were a failure or a Nobel Prize winner, we are all in the same boat. Of course, the same boat is being old, being eightysomething. It is the current day that matters.

When I began my interviews for this book, I assumed everyone would want to talk about their memories. But I was surprised to find it wasn't so. Beryl, a dynamo of a woman living in California, dismissed my question about her past by saying, "I don't dwell in the past. I am too busy to look back." The majority of the people said more or less the same thing—they just don't think all that much about their past.

They also expressed few regrets overall. Several people did admit that they wished they had gone back to school or changed careers. A few had regrets about getting divorced, and some wished they had gotten divorced sooner. But the vast majority have made their peace with the ups and downs of their lives and spend little time rehashing the past.

According to recent research, people who perceive that they have lots of opportunity to make changes in the future express more regrets than those with fewer opportunities.[1] Obviously, eightysomethings perceive they have little time to redo earlier decisions. It's too late for a different college, a different career, more children. No point in crying over spilt milk. No point focusing on what can't be changed. Fewer regrets than when they were younger.

There were, however, among those I interviewed, a few people whose regrets were still causing them pain in their eighties. Some of these with painful regrets were those who had experienced the death of a child. Verna, eighty-eight, for example, is one who still mourns every day the death of her five-year-old son over fifty years ago. In the first ten minutes of our interview, she mentioned his death and told me how it happened. He had suddenly spiked a high fever while they were on a family camping trip in Idaho. She wishes she had gotten him to a doctor sooner.

There are reasons people don't get over the death of a small child. A parent's love for a child is almost always unconditional, meaning that our love for our young children is often the strongest emotion we will ever feel, even stronger than the love for our mate. The loss of such a beloved child, with all their promise in front of them, makes the loss uniquely hard to accept.

If most eightysomethings have few regrets and don't talk much about their past, it is paradoxical that many of them begin to spend time reflecting on their lives. Often they decide to write about their past. Some sign up for a memoir class. The oldest eightysomethings, particularly the few surviving World War II veterans, want to capture their experiences. And even those who were just small children during the war recall the special feelings of that time and write about them.

Many eightysomethings enjoy writing about their childhood. They find it a great pleasure to remember their early years—the happy times, the adventures, the challenges. Their adult years are somewhat different. Most eightysomethings were so busy with their work and families during those years that their memories are a hazy blur. And they have less desire to write about those decades.

A few eightysomethings are storytellers and do talk about the past with their families. Sometimes their stories are loved by the family. But sometimes the younger generation isn't interested in grandpa's or grandma's stories. Sometimes their reaction is, "Oh, no, grandpa is going to tell that stupid story again."

If being eightysomething means your past is by definition long and complicated, it also means that your future is vastly diminished. They know that time is running out. As famous Yankee catcher Yogi Berra said, "The future ain't what it used to be."

Beryl, who blew off my questions about the past, also dismissed my question about the future just as quickly. "The future will take care of itself," she announced with authority. Beryl looks like the archetypal grandmother. She has a round face set off by a halo of white curls. Her body is rounded, too, and she moves with ease. She has lived with a woman friend for more than twenty-five years, and they moved to a retirement village in southern California about five years ago. She continued, "I don't do much planning for the future. I am taking a cruise next summer, but that is as far out as I can think." Then, as an after-thought she added, "I only worry that if I were to die, who would take care of Marta?"

About her daily life at home, Beryl said, "I live in the present. I do a little of this and a little of that, including five games of Scrabble on the computer each day with a daughter, and taking two beagles out for at least two walks." She spends hours preparing for the three courses she teaches for twelve weeks twice a year at her retirement community. When I spoke with her, the subjects were Native Americans in California, the Islamic Golden Age, and European Lives, 1715–1914. She is also doing research about a family member who experienced a shipwreck. She asks herself each day, "What new thing have I learned today?"

Beryl is clearly an outlier in the cohort of eightysomethings in terms of her energy, lack of memory loss, good health, financial resources, and freedom. Her focus on the present and her optimistic attitude contribute to her productivity and zest. She doesn't even notice that she is proving wrong all the stereotypes about what eighty-year-olds can and can't do.

Most eightysomethings have much quieter lives than Beryl, like Herb. Herb at eighty-five no longer does much. Like Beryl, though, he says he lives in the present. And what interests me about him are the changes in his attitude that he reported.

Herb was an urologist living in New York before he retired to southern California almost twenty years ago. He is a slight man, all skin and bones, with piercing black eyes. He had fun being interviewed—he enjoyed having me as a captive audience, so he could make a series of little speeches. Herb explained about his Parkinson's: "It gets in the way of everything. What used to take me one minute, takes me eight now. I can't email anymore, can't use the computer really. This last year I broke two hips but I can get around with a walker."

Herb admits he used to be impatient and short with people back when he was practicing medicine. Even ten years ago he used to bark at the staff at his retirement facility. He said,

> As I became more disabled, I had to change or just be miserable
> all the time. I am more Buddhist, letting go of trying to hurry
> and get things done. I don't get angry anymore—it is no longer

part of my makeup. I am more tolerant of others' mistakes. I got rid of my own "shoulds" and "ought tos." The key to how I live now is that I am not afraid. I go places. I socialize a lot. I come to life in a group. Many days I eat lunch with friends, and every dinner I eat with my girlfriend and friends. Of course, I take a lot of naps, too.

The future? I don't plan ahead because of my illness. I don't talk two years ahead, one year ahead. I really am living in the moment, curious about what the next moment will be. I don't look backward. What do I worry about? What is for dinner?

I have no need to do anything and I am not responsible for anything. I don't worry about the grandchildren like I used to. I gave up trying to influence their behavior. They live in such another world. Let them be who they are. They are going to live their lives anyway. I can't give advice anymore. But I can't help wondering, if my health were good, would I still be an interfering person?

Letty, eighty-four, unlike Herb, experiences herself as basically unchanged since she was young and contracted polio. She looks youthful, with short, straight brown hair. She radiates calm despite the fact that she is in a wheelchair and the world around her is changing week by week. Her husband, Dave, has advanced dementia. Letty said, "We have a limited future because of that. Already there are so many things he can't do. Recently I have taken over the finances and do all the driving. But I like to think that maybe I have another good decade in me."

She continued,

> At twenty-two, I contracted polio and my legs became paralyzed. I was despairing, almost without hope. My doctor was so mean to me that I became angry with him and I learned how

to become a fighter. I learned to walk again, too, although I am now back in a wheelchair much of the time. But I have never been depressed again.

My mission now is all about the family. I take care of Dave and I know there is an important role for me as a grandparent. I invited the kids and their spouses and grandkids to come for Christmas. If I hadn't invited them, the grandchildren wouldn't see each other since they live far apart. I encourage them not to put things off and to do lots of athletic things like skiing and hiking, things that they can't do forever.

Beryl, Herb, and Letty are people who have all found ways to be happy in their present circumstances—without many regrets or plans for the future. In my view, Beryl, the eightysomething Wonder Woman, feels like she is fifty. I wonder if she will be able to adapt when the time comes that she herself needs help. She has had so little practice in receiving, and so many successes.

Herb, now that he has given up trying to control others, is happier than he could have imagined. He seems to have figured out how to live in the now, the present moment. What an achievement to live without fear! Letty has her mission, trying to hold her family together. Her internal strength makes me feel confident that she will manage whatever lies ahead with competence and heart.

Most eightysomethings, like Beryl, don't make plans further out than eighteen months. Even though statistically, if you make it to eighty you will live, on average, for eight more years, none of those I spoke with were comfortable making plans that far ahead. This sense of uncertainty about the future is universal. They just can't count on being in good shape two years hence.

The uncertainty makes eightysomethings ambivalent about upcoming events like a family wedding or graduation. On the one hand, it is anticipated with great pleasure. On the other hand, it can be a source of worry at the same time. What happens if they fall? Or get sick and ruin things for everyone? They certainly don't want to be a burden on anyone. And some of those who are frail or fearful will decide not to go to the event at all.

Eightysomethings feel the world of technology is galloping along at such a breakneck pace that they have no hope of keeping up. The future seems more and more to be a place that they will not fit in. Each year they fall further behind. It doesn't really help them to feel better when their children or even their grandchildren say they can't keep up either. Most are satisfied with what they can do—emails, games, the Internet, movies, reading or watching the news, reading books, and listening. All but three or four of those I interviewed use email.

Even knowing that their own future is bound to be limited, some eightysomethings continue to work to leave the world a better place. They plant trees knowing they will not see them bear fruit. They are actively involved in all sorts of causes to save the planet and help eliminate poverty. They think long and hard about which organizations to support, and they vote carefully and often.

Most eightysomethings no longer have a bucket list of things they must do or places they must go before they die. When I last spoke to Mimi, my high school classmate, she told me she had just returned from Sri Lanka. That was the last item on her bucket list. Her last big trip. She said the need to go had been greater than her fear of falling. She was the one who had amazed us all when she had parachuted out of a plane when she turned fifty. I felt sad that Mimi wouldn't be traveling any more. She had always been an inspiration for me facing the world so fearlessly.

I, like most other eightysomethings, don't spend that much time thinking about my past or my future. I used to have a long list of regrets. I wished I had gone to Stanford because it was co-ed. I regretted that I majored in history rather than psychology. I regretted that I didn't start on my career before I turned thirty. I was sorry that John and I never had the opportunity to live outside the country for a whole year.

But somewhere, maybe when I turned eighty, maybe earlier, all those inner voices quieted down. I can hardly remember them. Today, I woke up at just before seven as the sunrise was beginning to paint the sky golden and pink. I lingered at the window, present for the amazing light show.

All of us, at all ages, are told we should live in the present. We are taught that the present moment is all there is. There is definitely something to learn from eightysomethings about how to live in the here and now. It is not a fountain of youth that can transform our lives to make them more joyful. Young people, with their beauty, health, strength, and capacity are usually struggling to figure out who they are and striving to make their place in the world. Paradoxically, eightysomethings with their many losses and multiple health issues find themselves naturally living in the present. And even better, they find themselves at peace.

CONVERSATION STARTERS

- How often do you spend time thinking about your past? What memories come often to you?
- What regrets do you have about past decisions? Have they faded over the years?
- What are your thoughts about your future? Hopes? Plans?
- When during your daily life is it that you feel most engaged? Most fully present?

TIPS FOR FAMILIES

- Tell your eightysomething that you would like to hear some stories about their life. Ask for memories from childhood, about their family, youthful adventures. Just listening is a huge gift.

- Or tell them you would like to interview them about their life. Some people need your questions to get going. The interview will mean a lot to them and to you and the grandchildren.
- Ask them about their pleasures in their life today. See how you can make them happen more often.
- Make a list with them of things they would like to do in the next year. This can bring focus and spice to their present life. See the list of "50 Exciting Things for Eightysomethings to Do" in Appendix I.

CHAPTER 11

DEMENTIA

On stage, an eightysomething woman and a youngish man were singing a duet, "You'll Never Walk Alone." The harmony was lovely, although the woman's voice wavered. It was the annual talent show at my retirement community. As the song came to a finish, the audience broke into thunderous applause and a standing ovation. Most of them knew the woman had advanced dementia and could no longer talk—but she can sing like an angel. And they knew the man beside her in the white suit was her aide at the Memory Unit where she lives. Many of those in the audience were in tears.

Among eightysomethings, nothing is dreaded more than dementia. When an eightysomething can't come up with a word or a name, which can happen many times in a day, they get flustered and upset. They routinely announce, "It's Alzheimer's." One person I interviewed told me she tells her family, "If I don't recognize any of you, please shoot me."

Most people of all ages, despite their fear of dementia, are not knowledgeable about Alzheimer's or dementia, so here are some facts. As of 2018 there are five million people in the United States living with dementia and this number will increase significantly as the Baby Boomers age. Nearly 50 percent of people over eighty-five will be diagnosed at some point with dementia.[1]

Many people do not know that dementia is the umbrella term and Alzheimer's, the most common form of dementia, accounts for 60 percent of the cases of dementia. Other dementias are vascular, temporal lobe, dementia with Lewy body, and Parkinson's dementia. Among patients at the 15,460 nursing homes in the United States, 42 percent are moderately or severely cognitively impaired and 24 percent are mildly impaired.

Most people, also, do not know how to distinguish between dementia and normal memory loss. The quick way to differentiate the two is that normal memory loss is when you lose your keys. Dementia is when you put the key in the freezer.

And most people haven't heard the good news that dementia rates in the United States are on the wane. Education, exercise, and good medical care are delaying the onset and the effects of all kinds of dementia. In 2000, the average age of diagnosis was 80.7 and just twelve years later it had changed to 82.7. However, these huge rates of dementia in old age are terrifying to the elderly. Researchers are seeking a cure for Alzheimer's but acknowledge that eradicating it is still a distant dream.[2]

I met with Hector Montesino, a certified dementia specialist in the Boston area, to learn about his perspective on care for people with dementia. His first comment and main point was, "We can't think of everyone with dementia as falling into one box. Each person needs to be treated differently." As I proceeded with my interviews of a number of people with dementia, I saw for myself how very different they were one from another.

Montesino believes that the most common mistake that is made in caring for people with dementia is overprotection. He told me, "We need to watch out for their safety but also we need to give them choices. Caregivers tend to give too many commands."

Gus, an eighty-seven-year-old man who walks with a cane, was wearing a black T-shirt that showed off the distinctive tattoo of a dragon on his right arm the day he was interviewed. He has been attending a day program on the north shore of Massachusetts for people with physical and cognitive challenges for three years. A few individuals pay privately for the program, but most, like Gus, are on Medicaid or Mass Health that provide insurance to those at the bottom of the economic ladder.

Gus looked at his boots as the interview began but warmed up as it got going. Asked what he enjoys about his life, he replied, "Music. I like country western music, Eddy Arnold. I have been listening to him for years. He picks me up . . . . I like two other country singers, but I can't remember their names. And my dog. He's a big fella and he thinks the world of me. His name is Jack, a German shepherd. I think more people ought to follow that line and have a pet. They bring out the best in me. My dog is very important to me. He barks at strangers."

When I asked about life as an eighty-year-old person, he said, "I am enjoying it. The freedom of not being penalized by anybody." Concerning what's hard in his life, he said, "It's hard to remember things, dates and things. It's not a good feeling. It's not scary, but I got to realize that. My boyhood, I can't remember anything at all about when I was young."

Gus is moderately cognitively impaired. He is able to live on his own and manage his life day-to-day with the help of his program. He knows he has memory problems and is bothered by them, while people with more advanced dementia are often are unaware of their dementia.

Prue, eighty-seven, like Gus, is able to talk about her memory loss. She lives on a farm with her husband in central Virginia. She has curly red-gray hair and velvety brown eyes. But most notable are the hundreds of freckles sprinkled over her face and arms. Long days in the sun, I thought when I met her.

Prue told me, "I can't remember who my friends are. I go into town and see somebody that seems familiar. So I tell them 'I know that I know you, but I can't remember your name. I have lost my memory.'" Later in the interview she admitted to me how jealous she is of her husband, Jim, who can meet new people and remember their names. And he can still travel and likes gatherings, while she is finding them increasingly difficult. She said, "But I still do care how I look." Prue spends her time talking to her children on the phone and listening around the clock to National Public Radio.

I am astonished at how emotionally savvy Prue is despite her cognitive impairment. She is aware of her memory slipping away from her and has developed coping skills to handle this. She retains a gracious personality and a sense of self and wholeness, despite her losses.

Maddie's dementia is more advanced than Prue's but, like her, she has retained some of her social skills. Maddie, eighty-six, lives in the independent living section of a retirement community near Boston, but she stays in her apartment almost all of the time. On the day I met with her at eleven in the morning she was wearing a rumpled pink robe and a flowery nightgown. Her gray hair was a bit messy, but her smile was friendly.

Maddie reported that the arthritis in her feet was particularly bad that day and that she had not felt up to going to the lobby to get her usual cup of coffee. Her kids, she explained, have given her several types of coffee-makers, but she can't figure out how to use them.

I'd told her that I wanted to talk about her daily life. She began with, "I have big time memory loss. The memory situation is totally weird. So I just go with the flow. If I don't remember, I don't remember. I'm that kind of person. I came with social skills. And I have a boyfriend. That is pretty darn nice at this age. I have dinner with him most nights. He is getting a little iffy in his head and he doesn't remember a lot of things. He looks fragile and thin. But he can manage his life."

Maddie didn't know how long she has lived in her apartment or where she went for Thanksgiving. But her long-term memory, as is common for those with dementia, is still somewhat intact. And, she had lots to say about her life. She said her pleasures are getting up when she wants. Doing what she wants. When she came to the retirement community, she did not want to be on any committees, didn't want any responsibilities. "From time to time, I do step in and try to be helpful. I like to talk to people," she said. She told me she has the TV on most of the time. "I don't know what they are saying—it's company."

Maddie continued, "I am lucky to be healthy except for my back and the arthritis in my feet. I have fallen a number of times. But I don't tell anybody. I don't much believe in doctors. One time a year is plenty. It is fine for me here in this apartment in this place. I don't have to go anywhere. I have nature right outside to look at," she said, gesturing at the green trees outside her window. "But there is a lot of stuff you can't fix. A lot you have no control over, so you step aside. And life settles out."

Russell lives in a large retirement complex south of Boston. Compared to Maddie, Russell is a man of few words. His wife had answered the phone when I called to arrange the interview. She explained that Russell has memory loss but is comfortable talking about it. I told her that is wonderful since I am interested in hearing what his life is like from the perspective of people with memory loss.

The day we met, Russell was wearing brown corduroy pants and a maroon crew neck sweater. He is a lanky, handsome man with a slightly dazed expression. When I asked him about his daily life and what gives him pleasure, he was stumped. After a very long pause he went right to his memory problems. "I have lived so long, had so much in my mind, it is inevitable that I have forgotten a lot. I couldn't hold it all in." After another minute, he told me that he enjoys playing the piano and reading. At that point, his wife called in from the next room, "Russell also enjoys jigsaw puzzles, crossword puzzles, and suduko." Russell responded, "And I have an understanding wife who helps, no, who fills in occasionally, for me." I looked up and his wife had slipped into the room and joined the interview.

Russell went on to say that he likes the retirement community where they live and is glad he has no commitments. It is a pleasant life. He told me, "I don't worry because I am well-assisted." His wife added that they decide together what they will do each day. "As long as I remind him, he can do most things."

Russell can do most things because he has a wife who can speak for him when he has trouble finding words. She not only speaks for him, she navigates the world for him, plans for him, and cares for him. He is right; he has is well-assisted and I am glad he finds it a pleasant life.

Of course, living with dementia is not always pleasant, especially as the disease progresses. There is often emotional deregulation, continual loss of cognitive abilities, self-awareness, and ability to relate. Not only do people with dementia lose their connection with their loved one, but they also require years of backbreaking care, often provided by a spouse.

For example, as I left Russell's apartment, I found myself sharing an elevator with a woman and her aide. The woman was screaming at her aide, saying over and over, "You are bad. You are bad. You are bad." I was unsettled, wanting to calm the woman who apparently had dementia and, even more, I wanted to comfort the aide. But, before I could figure out what to say, they exited at the next floor. I was left with a knot of pain in my stomach.

Carl, eighty-nine, is a former executive, who lives at a retirement complex south of Philadelphia that includes a nursing home, an assisted living section, and a memory unit. Carl's wife, Maud, had been diagnosed with Alzheimer's fifteen years ago and has been living in the memory unit for twelve years. She hasn't recognized him for at least nine years and doesn't speak. I interviewed Carl to learn about the long-term impact of her Alzheimer's on him and her family. He is a soft-spoken, gentle man. He prepared some notes for our interview and seemed to be glad to be telling his story.

At first, when Maud was diagnosed, Carl worried that people might blame her illness on him. Would they think he had caused it in some way? In the early days of her impairment, he felt "stupid and inadequate" when he couldn't persuade her to take her medicine or do what the doctor wanted. He didn't know how to handle several doctors who were quite insensitive to his wife. It took a few false moves to get the right care for her.

One day Maud couldn't remember how to turn the car on. Carl had wondered months before if she should continue driving, but he didn't know how to stop her. Then as Maud's condition worsened, he realized it was no longer safe for Maud to be alone in the house, and they needed to move. After several years in the retirement community, as Maud's disease progressed, it became time for her to move into a memory unit. Carl couldn't care for her any longer. For a number of years, he visited at the memory unit three or four times a week, checking on her health and her care. Their three children usually came from time to time, as well.

"Then," Carl continued, "there was a stage where Maud became hostile." One day as he leaned over to kiss her hello, she bit his cheek so badly he had to go to the emergency room. And she kicked a lot during that time. "The angry stage passed but then as the months passed, Maud couldn't talk, walk, or feed herself. Today the only movement she makes is to open her mouth when she is being fed. But she is healthy."

Carl has realized that she may well outlive him, as "She rarely gets a cold." He visits her less often now and so do the kids. He has no sense that his visits mean anything to her: she shows no acknowledgment that he is there. "But I don't think she suffers." he said. Yet, he still feels guilty that he doesn't visit more often.

Carl says that looking back he did do some things right. "First, I never tried to hide her illness from the kids. We were a family team making decisions together at each stage of her disease." And he was lucky because he had the money to hire help. Secondly, he has always tried to be kind. They had many aides; some of them Maud liked and some she didn't. He has been lucky and one of them, a lovely woman from Uganda, has been with Maud for many years.

Maud's dementia, he acknowledged, has taken a devastating toll on the family. The two daughters, in particular, have missed having a mother all these years. But on the positive side, they all have memories of the good years. He added, "Alzheimer's is not the worst disease in the world because self-awareness is destroyed as it progresses. When you know what is going on, that is far worse." He thinks his kids are probably worried that Alzheimer's is in their genes. But he hasn't talked about it with them and he hasn't done any research to find out to what degree the disease does run in families.

Carl's story is typical of many families trying to cope with Alzheimer's. At the start, they deny what is going on. As the disease progresses, they don't know how to take control or set limits on a formerly independent person. They feel guilty. Finally, they learn to accept what is and what they need to do to adapt to the gradual deterioration of their loved one.

Lack of information breeds fear. And the media often portrays people with dementia with negative images and language. Terms like the "long goodbye" and "war against" evoke a sense of impending tragedy. Challenging negative perceptions and creating more meaningful programs of engagement that support the mind, body, and spirit are needed.

ARTZ (Artists for Alzheimer's), a nonprofit foundation based in Woburn, Massachusetts, has done groundbreaking work using the arts and cultural inclusion to improve the lives of those with dementia. In 2010, ARTZ created the first museum programs for people with Alzheimer's at the Museum of Modern Art in New York City. Today, museum programs for older adults with memory loss have sprung up throughout the United States as well as internationally.

While attending an art program for people with dementia at a local museum and exploring some beautiful watercolors, Carol Ann, who lives at a nursing home, said, "This is great. It's like coming alive. I could do this all day."

Gus, who attended another program, decorated a lantern with painted rice paper. When he finished, he said, "This is my pride and joy."

Peggy Cahill, a community educator who has been creating arts and culture programs for people with dementia in Maine and Massachusetts, believes there is much work yet to be done to lessen the stigma of dementia and preserve the dignity of those who have it. And, she said, eightysomethings with dementia face double stigmatization—their dementia plus their age. She told me, "If we cannot provide quality of life, extending life through medical intervention is not the answer. We must make a life worth living for people with dementia." Many nursing homes, however, do not have the resources to provide these kinds of arts and culture programs. Understaffing, low salaries, and high turnover rates leaves staff with little time to explore an individual's unique history, needs, and passions.

From my interviews, I experienced over and over that beyond the cognitive loss in a person with dementia, there remains a multi-dimensional human being, a soul. They all have their own style, their stories, their complicated past life, and their struggles to cope with memory loss. Perhaps more than any other group of eightysomethings, they have been stigmatized and made invisible in our society. There is still so much work to do to create environments where all people with dementia are treated with the dignity they deserve.

CONVERSATION STARTERS
- What are you enjoying most in your life nowadays?
- What is hard for you in your life right now? What helps?
- What do you do when you can't remember something?
- Do you try to keep your family from knowing about your difficulties or do you tell them about them?

TIPS FOR FAMILIES
- When dealing with someone with dementia, remember their long-term memory may well be intact.

- Provide choices but keep them simple—two alternatives is enough.
- If your eightysomething seems to have significant memory loss, talk to their doctor about it.
- Read *The 36-Hour Day* by Nancy L. Mace. It is wonderful book to read to learn more about dementia and Alzheimer's.

CHAPTER 12

TRANSITIONS

A transition is different from a change, according to William Bridges, author of the bestselling book *Transitions: Making Sense Out of Life's Changes*. He describes transitions as having three phases: "an *ending* that is the beginning, an *in-between time* that can feel like being lost and wandering in the wilderness, and, finally, a *new beginning*. It involves external events but it is more than that; it also involves an inner reorientation and revised sense of identity. It requires a psychological process of evolution."[1]

All transitions are stressful and disruptive to some degree. Even happy ones like a marriage are stressful because they all involve loss, the loss of a former way of life. Fifty years ago, psychiatrists Thomas Holmes and Richard Rahe developed a scale that assigns points for amount of stress caused by various life events. The death of a spouse is the most stressful item on their scale, at 100 points. Other major stressors include divorce, getting fired, marriage, a diagnosis of a major medical problem, and moving. The theory is that, whenever people are in the midst of a number of transitions simultaneously, their cumulative stress points are at such a high level that they are likely to become ill.[2]

Unlike transitions in earlier life stages, which are typically sought, late-life transitions are usually faced with reluctance and foot dragging. Moving from one home to another is one of most common transitions that people experience in their eighties. Other frequent transitions encountered are giving up driving, needing to use a walker, or spending time in a hospital. All these transitions are usually difficult. They not only require changes in lifestyle but also can diminish self-confidence and self-esteem.

Moving from their home of many years is a transition that the vast majority of people in their eighties want to avoid. They make Herculean efforts to prove to themselves and their families that they can manage in their old home.

Most eightysomethings are successful in staying put: at age eighty-five, 70 percent of them are living in their own homes.[3] That means, of course, that 30 percent are living in other kinds of places. They move from their homes of many years to smaller homes, to live with their children, to condos and senior apartments, to retirement communities, and to skilled nursing facilities. As their health declines, eightysomethings often go back and forth to the hospital numbers of times.

Avery's move from her home of many years illustrates the process of an eightysomething move in slow motion. It highlights many of the kinds of issues that can arise. Avery, eighty-three, was a freelance writer whose last full-time job was when she was twenty-six. Forty years ago, she and her husband, Nat, moved to a house in a large city in Virginia.

Avery, who is willowy and still beautiful, flutters with nervous energy. As we talked, she stood up and sat down several times. Nat's death, seven years ago, was the triggering event leading to her eventual move. She remembered she felt panicky right from the start because Nat had done all the house maintenance inside and out.

The first year Avery let the garden go. The next year she had to deal with a leaky roof and clogged gutters, and then it was water in the basement. Then Avery began to feel out of place in the neighborhood among all the young parents with their baby carriages and dogs. While people treated her with politeness, she believed they were just making nice to an old lady. Her inner voice was relentless: *It is time to move and the house is obviously too much to handle.* But to decide to sell the house was not doable. She told me, "I knew I was dithering, but I couldn't stop."

About the fourth year after Nat died, Avery met Tyler on Match.com. Soon he was coming to visit her most weekends and sometimes he stayed over for a week or so. He wasn't much help with the house, though, because of neuropathy in his legs and other medical conditions. A year later, they decided it made sense to move together to a retirement community. They selected a continuing care senior facility, where they thought they would fit in.

Avery was glad that the decision to move was finally made. In terms of Bridges' language, the first phase of her transition had been accomplished. Now in the in-between phase, she felt anxious, untethered, and lost.

Avery and Tyler went for their formal medical appointments at the facility. Two weeks later they got a call saying that, because Tyler's medical problems were significant, they would not be offering him a contract to live there. According to Avery, the people at the facility said the doctor believed that Tyler had Parkinson's. Tyler was crushed. His rejection was a devastating blow to Avery, too. It cast a pall over the whole idea of a move and, it seems, over their relationship, as well.

Tyler decided to return to his home in Maryland. Avery used this unexpected derailment of their plans to rethink where she really wanted to go as well to reevaluate her relationship with Tyler. After some weeks, she decided to continue the search for a place to move on her own; she realized she did not want Tyler to be her life partner.

It was a huge relief to Avery when several friends who lived in a senior apartment building right in the city urged her to move there. That felt like a solution she could accept. Naturally, there was more indecision, as she considered five different apartments in the new building as they became available. Each one had issues—one was too dark, another too small. But at last, she found one that worked for her.

Avery's two children and their spouses came several weekends and helped her clear out the house. But she told them not to come on moving day, as she would be perfectly fine without them. She hired a friend who had a moving business to help her. On moving day her friend took over completely—telling the movers what to do and where things went. Avery lamented, "I just walked aimlessly here and there, feeling forlorn and side-lined. The whole day was sad for me."

After the move, in her new apartment, Avery still didn't feel quite like herself. She was slow to unpack all the boxes and had difficulties deciding where things should go. But she felt comfortable just knowing friends were in the building. It was four months, however, before she was ready to invite any friends over. When she did, that dinner was a milestone for her. It was the moment she finally felt she was at home. She continues to talk to Tyler on the phone, but since he doesn't drive, they rarely see each other.

This saga illustrates just how hard transitions can be when you are in your eighties. Avery's difficulties getting in touch with what she really wanted stretched her moving process out by years. It was a long period of confusion. It is important to realize that during these long periods where apparently no progress was being made, Avery was mourning the loss of her home and letting go of her old lifestyle. It often takes time to achieve the inner readiness to actually move. Then in Avery's case, she had a sec-ond loss to grieve when the possibility of a new life with Tyler melted away as she decided she did not want him as her life partner.

Another important issue in Avery's story is her unrealistic assessment of her abilities. She sent out the message that she could go it alone, but that was mostly bravado. Inside, she felt fragile, dependent, and insecure. She couldn't accept help easily, and when she did get help it made her uneasy. And, lastly, her image of what it meant to be old remains very negative. In her mind, younger people would not want to be with an "old lady" like her.

My own move to a retirement facility, like Avery's, was also painful, though it was accomplished far more quickly. The ending began when John told me he felt unable to do all the maintenance that our home of twenty-five years required. He needed to move. He was eighty-two and I was seventy-six. I agreed that it was better for us, as a couple, to move. I was more dubious about me. I hoped I could continue my life—my private practice, my writing group, my church, my friendships—by moving to the retirement community right in our town. Nothing would have to change. In three months, we were settled in our new apartment.

The hard part came after the move. I felt I didn't belong in the place with so many older people. I was one of the very few who was still working. When people kept telling me how fast I walked, I felt it was said with resentment and not friendliness. I just quietly became more and more depressed. My funk lasted at least a year; some of my friends say it was two years. Since I am not one to complain, I would tell people I was soooo happy in our new home while inside I was hurting.

In my case, all my knowledge and training as a psychotherapist didn't help at all. What did help was working and still having clients who valued my skills. Over time I made new friends. Finally, I could honestly say I was happy and mean it. I was ready to admit that I, too, was old, not some exception to aging just because I was still working and could do push-ups. And now that I am eighty-four, and a widow, the fit is even better.

Virginia's experience, so different from both Avery's and mine, was an easy transition and a happy one. She had been on her own for decades, as her husband died twenty-five years ago. Virginia is a soft-spoken, gentle woman who ran a gift shop for twenty years. She told me, "Moving shakes you up in a good way if you are not afraid of new experiences. I usually welcome change. When I went on a trip alone a few years ago, I decided not to go to Florida where I had already been several times, but to go to the Grand Canyon."

Before her move, Virginia was living in an apartment that was cold and impersonal. The only older women in the building played mahjong all day. From the first day at a residential retirement community near Boston, she loved being there: "The architecture welcomes—it has an open and sunny lobby, and now, after a year of being here, I feel surrounded by friends. When I come through the door, I usually meet three people. I'll stop and talk for a minute. There is a lovely community spirit."

After a month at the community, Virginia, now eighty-three, met a man named Brad and they began *seeing* each other. (That is the wording used at the community when new couples form.) It all happened quickly and they decided to keep it under the radar for a few months because Brad's wife had died recently.

Of course, said Virginia, "Dealing with aging looms large in my life." She took a course last year on aging wisely that met once a week for eight weeks. "Just the fact going to the class helped me to face my aging, I could no longer ignore it. Now, I see aging as a challenge, like climbing a mountain. It helped me see the move as a challenge, too, and made my move so easy."

It wasn't just luck that made Virginia's move such a pleasant one; it was her attitude of embracing change. Of course, because she was friendly herself, she attracted people to her right away. She felt like she was part of the community in a matter of days. Feeling you belong and are part of a community is a key to happiness in one's eighties. Of course, it must be said that Virginia had the good sense to realize she would be happier in a community and to move. In general, I believe Americans put too much emphasis on the importance of independence and staying in their own home even when they will be isolated and lonely. We are social animals and we thrive when we are in community.

Julianne, whose husband died a year ago, has found the transition to life on her own an ongoing struggle. This is not surprising since the death of a spouse is for most people the most stressful of all transitions. It can mean the loss of the love of their life, their best friend, their mooring, their day-to-day job, their counselor. The death of a spouse also brings the loss of role, status, and identity as a husband or wife. They are now a widower or widow. They are no longer a "we."

But each situation is different, and Julianne's story of the death of her husband, Ian, is no fairy tale. She began, "When Ian died suddenly after being ill for several years, I had a mix of emotions and finally came to grips with the reality that we didn't have a good marriage. I was concerned that I couldn't be the adoring weeping widow that is expected. In fact, I wasn't sure I would ever grieve at all. So when tears did arrive after several days, I felt relieved."

Julianne, eighty-one, gathered steam as she got into her story. When she was in her mid-fifties, she found hundreds of emails on Ian's computer from another woman. They were loving and intimate. It was an ongoing affair. Ian admitted there had been a series of other women going back decades. Julianne was devastated and angry. She felt Ian was a "complete scumbag" and in a few weeks asked him to leave the house. He refused, so Julianne moved out herself and found a nearby apartment. To her surprise she loved the apartment and how free and happy she felt.

But Julianne felt it was too late for her to start a complete new life and soon she and Ian began getting together for weekends. They had wonderful friends and many good times, but Julianne found her heart wasn't in the marriage anymore: "I had a battle inside me, I wanted to do what I wanted to do. The marriage limped along as a part-time arrangement." In their late seventies, they sold their house, Julianne gave up the apartment she had held onto for almost thirty years, and they moved to the retirement community in Connecticut, close to New Haven where one of their daughters lives.

Two years ago Ian got sick and, at that point, Julianne became a full-time caregiver. They couldn't afford to hire anyone, so for those two years she never left their apartment except for a few hours a week when her daughter took over. Ian's death was a shock, a blessing, and a relief. She was still angry, and she still loved him.

It has taken Julianne a long time to deal with all the practical aspects of Ian's death. Her daughter helped in planning the memorial service and continues to help in many ways from paying the bills to going to doctor's appointments with Julianne. Julianne tells me she is grateful for her daughter. But she admits she doesn't really feel in charge of her life because her daughter does so much. Julianne is not back to being herself; she is not even sure what that would mean—herself before Ian was sick, herself before she learned of all the affairs, or herself before he died?

Clearly this is a situation of complicated grief. Grieving is always more difficult when there are feelings of anger that have never been fully resolved. Julianne and Ian never worked through their issues enough to either make a new commitment to each other or to separate for good. She is also bothered by her daughter doing so much for her. As I see it, her upset is not really about her daughter. Rather it is about Julianne struggling to take control of her life once again. When I interviewed her it was just eight months after Ian's death and she was still wandering in the wilderness. Not yet ready to start planning for a new day and not yet exploring new possibilities. With more time, perhaps she will find a way to feel free and happy once again.

The transitions that eightysomethings experience can be difficult at every stage along the way, as can be seen from the stories of Avery and Julianne, and from my experience, too. Yet, transitions can sometimes be easy, like Virginia's.

Perhaps the most difficult part of a transition is the inner, unseen transition that has to take place in order to adjust to new and different circumstances. Avery needed to become aware she did not want to be Tyler's partner or to move into a retirement community before she could make the decision to move from her house. I needed to change my sense of myself and accept that I, too, was old in order to flourish at my retirement community. Albert Einstein said, "The world we have created is a product of our thinking. It cannot be changed without changing our thinking." But that part of life transitions often goes unrecognized.

CONVERSATION STARTERS

- What big transition have you been through in your eighties? What was it like for you?
- What helped you adapt to the new place or role? What hindered your adjustment?
- How did your inner sense of yourself evolve after a big transition?
- Is there another transition on the horizon, a transition that you feel you need to make?

TIPS FOR FAMILIES

- Sometimes adult children need to make the hard call when it is time for an eightysomething to move or go to the hospital, but in most cases your role should be to help them make the right call themselves.
- Family members can provide much-needed help with the mountain of tasks a move requires or with the tasks that follow a death. Remember, though, that it is just as important to stop doing and listen. Let your elderly parents mourn the losses that a transition means for them.
- Remember that the pace of getting things done by people in their eighties may be far slower that what you expect. They may need to take their time.
- Some adult children provide too much help, more than an eightysomething wants or needs. Ask them directly if they want less help, more help, or the same amount of help you're already providing.

CHAPTER 13

SURVIVOR SKILLS

Each one of today's almost ten million octogenarians in the United States is a survivor. They are the lucky ones. Half of the people in their original cohort have died. But three fourths of them live on incomes that are less than twenty thousand dollars per year.[1] And many of them contend with medical conditions.

Life as an eightysomething is, therefore, more challenging for people than when they were younger. Yet, somehow, eightysomethings cope. Those at the low end of the economic ladder have learned how to make do with smaller incomes. Those with medical problems have adapted to their disabilities. And those who have lost spouses, family members, and friends have learned how to grieve their losses and keep on going.

Pindar, who lived into his eighties in fifth century BC, wrote about how to age well. He said, "Do not aspire for immortality, but exhaust the realm of the possible."[2] And people in their eighties today are people who have explored the realm of the possible. The stories of Miguel, Jackie, Mazelle, Denny, and Claude show how ordinary people in their eighties develop skills to keep on surviving.

Miguel, eighty-two, has to count every penny. I met him for coffee at a cafe near his home in Worcester, west of Boston. He is a tallish, slightly overweight man wearing jeans, a T-shirt, and a baseball cap pulled low.

The first thing Miguel told me was that both his parents were immigrants coming from Portugal as young people. He grew up in Fall River, Massachusetts, a blue-collar city, and began playing the trumpet in a

Portuguese band with his uncles when he was only ten years old. At seventeen, he went to work at a factory where his dad was working making nuts and bolts. When he was twenty, someone told him there was a music program at the local community college that he could probably get into. He did get in, and after graduation became a music teacher at a large high school. He retired at sixty-two, about twenty years ago.

Miguel and his second wife live on forty thousand dollars a year, pooling his pension from the state and her social security check. They are still paying a mortgage on their house, but he doesn't worry about money because his income is reliable, and he is not extravagant. They don't spend money on going out to eat or traveling.

I asked him how he has been able to live so long. "It's all luck," he replied. But then he told me that he has never smoked or done drugs. He keeps active, does work around the yard, and exercises three times a week. He has fun too, playing in a band every now and then with his old buddies. They love to perform Frank Sinatra songs. Miguel added, "The secret of my long life is naps. Every day at about 4:30, I take half a Valium and then sleep. I wake up refreshed and ready for the second half of my day."

Miguel said he gets along with all his family. He takes care of a five-year-old granddaughter once a week. "There is a calmness in my family—different from some families, and that calmness is part of what keeps me alive. I do not overreact to people. There is a lot of nastiness out there." He said he is not at all competitive. "I don't play to win. In fact, I like to play basketball by myself. I don't want anyone blocking my shots."

In my view, the fact that Miguel survives is not just good luck, although, for sure, anyone who sees an eightieth birthday has had much good fortune over many years. What I see as key for Miguel is his skill in self-management. He has chosen a healthy lifestyle, a life of moderation and restraint. It is his thousands of small choices that have made his survival more likely.

But Miguel also cultivates good relationships with his extended family and his buddies, avoiding overreaction, conflicts, and competition. Then we have his daily nap that he thinks is so important. Maybe he is right, it is as simple as that. The secret to a long life is a daily nap!

Jackie, eighty-three, is another eightysomething who lives with limited resources. I first met Jackie at a community dinner at a soup kitchen, near Boston. She and her husband were introduced to me as regulars, who come every Wednesday for the meal and to pick up a bag of groceries. She stood out in the group with her dyed bright golden hair, magenta lipstick, and powdery, pink cheeks. A few weeks later I met with her at their small apartment in her town's low-cost housing project.

Jackie remembered me from the soup kitchen and told me how many really nice people they have met there. She and her husband came down to Massachusetts from Maine ten years ago when they ran out of money. For four years their daughter took them in while they waited for their names to rise to the top of the list for an affordable apartment.

Jackie and her husband have impressive skills at surviving with little income. First, they had the organizational know-how to get their name on the right list for affordable housing. And it takes skill to find out where there is free food at a soup kitchen in a town twenty miles away.

Jackie used to think getting old would be terrible, with nothing to do. But her current life, she explained, has been full of pleasant surprises, particularly that she is just as busy as always. But since she has had two bad falls, she rarely goes out except for the community dinners and church. She said, "Money is always a concern but so far it hasn't overtaken us. We can do anything we want. I do crafts, though I haven't done much recently."

Jackie has embraced a positive attitude, saying she can do anything she wants. But I see that clearly this is not true. She is very limited after her falls; in fact, she can hardly walk. Her arthritis makes crafts impossible. Yet she sees her glass as full when she could more easily conclude it is half empty. Unlike Miguel, who lives an intentional life, Jackie does not appear to reflect much about her life. Being optimistic, however, has many benefits. And although I usually help my clients to be realistic in their thinking, it is different for Jackie. She shows us how, at times, denial can be useful as a coping skill. It works for her.

Mazelle, eighty-six, like Jackie, moved in with a daughter when she had no money and, like her, is optimistic about herself today. But what stood out for me about Mazelle was how she has learned to rebound from setbacks. Mazelle, an African-American woman, lives in west Philadelphia in a multigenerational household that also includes two of her daughters and a granddaughter. When I talked with her, Mazelle was sitting in a beat-up recliner with a crocheted quilt over her lap. Her fluffy gray hair and huge glasses gave her the look of a relaxed owl. After years of procrastinating, six weeks ago she finally took the plunge and had surgery to fix her knee. Beaming at me she said, "I am hopeful even though I have no plans. I am just enjoying myself now that I can walk again."

She told me,

> We all get on remarkably well in the house because we talk. If someone is misadjusted we have a family meeting. And if they are still misadjusted we have another meeting. My husband never talked much to me. I tried leaning on him but he wasn't stepping up to the plate, so I stopped. He wouldn't buy a house because his friends told him if you buy a house, she will put you out. He died twenty years ago. At first I thought "I am going to die because he died," but then I changed jobs, took some courses instead, and got a new job.
>
> After I retired, I had nowhere to go and I was depressed. That is when I came to live with my daughter. My bum leg was an excuse not to go anywhere and not to talk to anyone. I started to drink too much. First it was Harvey's Bristol Cream

and then on to vodka and Sprite. A therapist taught me to meditate. Although I stopped going to him, I was able to stop drinking. I don't know if it was the meditation or what.

Looking back, I haven't done very much in my life, but I feel I did all I could do. I took care of my mother. I would be exhausted but I would get up and care for her day after day. Now I want to do something, I might go to school for paralegals.

Mazelle is resilient and has developed the interpersonal skills to make living in a multigenerational family work well. She understands how talking helps. For the last few years she has been totally dependent on her family and has had to adapt to her loss of independence. Most important of all has been her ability to quit drinking. Alcoholics do not have longevity. Their lives are usually cut short way before they make it to eighty. Mazelle's idea of going back to school is probably unrealistic—but it reflects her new hopefulness now that she can walk again. While she doesn't feel she has accomplished much in her life, I see her ongoing growth and development over the years as no small achievement.

Denny, eighty-two, a cheerful Santa Claus of a man with the requisite pot belly and flowing white beard, is another person who was able to stop drinking. He told me, "Despite a rocky start and tough times, I am still alive and doing what I want—working for the union. I've had lucky breaks, too."

Denny and his wife live in Wisconsin on a mere twenty thousand dollars per year, half of Miguel's income. "The money is really okay," Denny assured me. "We buy the cheapest everything and drink no liquor. I read all the ads in the grocery stores and I save on everything. How come I survive? I never sit still. I have friends who spent all their days watching TV and they are no longer with us."

Denny left school after the eighth grade—a very bad decision, he said. He bummed around for a couple of years and then enlisted in the Navy for eight years. He married young and his wife promised to join him in Cuba where he was stationed. But she never arrived and he never heard from her again.

When he got out of the Navy, he got a good job at a large company in Wisconsin that makes industrial tools. Soon, however, he began drinking, and drinking too much. He would often call in sick after a late night and eventually he was fired. He was desperate. He went to his union for help and after several years, they were able to get the decision reversed. Denny not only got his job back, but he got all his back pay, too. "I was so grateful that I decided at that moment that I would spend the rest of my life working to promote unions. And I stopped drinking."

Denny married again and had four children. "But," he explained, "two of my kids died—one son had leukemia and the other committed suicide—he had been into drugs for years. It was a dark time. Today, things are so much better. My daughter is a chip off the old block and is active in the union and my other son lives right in town."

He continued, "Shortly after I retired, the company decided to stop honoring our pensions. The union fought this for decades, but finally the Supreme Court decided against us. It left me in bad shape."

For twenty-six years he was the head of his local chapter of union retirees. He was also president of Wisconsin's Alliance for Retired Americans and active with the Tincan Sailors—an organization of those who have served on destroyers. Then, because of his union work, he got to go to President Barack Obama's first inauguration in Washington, DC. He not only got to go there, but he also got a ticket to sit on the podium with all the big wigs like Madeleine Albright.

Today Denny has trouble walking because of his legs, and he has congestive heart failure. Despite his serious his health problems, he still keeps an amazing schedule for a man in his eighties.

Denny has developed many practical skills, so he can survive on an income that is below the poverty level. The fact that he had the willpower and grit to stop drinking is, of course, a huge key factor in Denny's being alive today. His dedication to supporting the union has given focus and meaning to his life for decades. Lastly, he is immersed in organizational activities and social activities connecting to a huge number of people every week.

Another important aspect of Denny's story that is not so obvious is that he has been able to cope with so many major losses over the years. He didn't get to finish high school, was abandoned by his first wife, lost his job, lost his pension, two children died, and now, in his eighties, he lives with the loss of much of the function of his heart.

Losses have the potential to overwhelm and derail a person at any age. People in their eighties can face an unending stream of losses, small and large. Perhaps that is the reason for the saying "old age is not for sissies." But it takes more than bravery to flourish in old age; it requires the ability to handle and accept, one by one, the losses that are encountered.

You may be asking, what exactly does it mean to handle, work through, and grieve a loss? The classic model of grieving that Elisabeth Kübler-Ross set forth years ago is still a useful place to start. She posits that the typical person dealing with a major loss moves through five emotional states: denial, anger, bargaining, depression, and acceptance.[3]

Denial usually comes first, a refusal to believe the loss has happened. And it can include both shock and numbness. Feeling angry typically comes next: "How can this happen to me?" "This is not fair," and, perhaps, cursing God or fate. Bargaining, the third stage, is when people make deals with the powers that be: "I will give up smoking, drinking, drugs, gambling, cheating if this turns out well." Depression, feeling down and hopeless, is the next stage. This can be fleeting and minor, or life changing and relentless. Lastly comes acceptance of the loss and the ability to move forward.

It is important to understand that not everyone goes through every stage in that order. People often cycle through each of the stages many times. Bargaining is frequently skipped over entirely. Handling a loss can be quick or it can take years. But when the emotional work of grieving is not done, a person can remain stuck in depression and unable to move on with living well. Though eightysomethings have all developed some skills to handle the losses that have come their way, many of them are not consciously aware of exactly how they do it. Some never complete their grief work.

Denny, it seems, is one who has handled his losses well enough to move on, though he can't put into words how he has done it. My view is that it has been his purpose in life—his work for the union—that has sustained him through loss and dark days. He has important work to do and a cause to which he is committed.

Claude, eighty-seven, a retired psychology and religious studies professor at a university in Texas, leads a far quieter life than Miguel, Jackie, Mazelle, and Denny, who all are busy. Claude reported, "I am not active, not out and about the campus, not writing. My wife has died, and I can't really walk more than a few feet. The riches in my life are the occasional visits from former students and faculty and enjoying my memories. I continue to focus on having conversations that matter. I seem, oddly, to be going a bit soft as I age. I find myself crying more than I have since I was a little boy."

Claude, a trim man who has a head of pure white hair and a pink, friendly face, was wearing a blue button-down shirt and sneakers in the photo I had of him. I learned that he had played an active role on campus during both the Civil Rights Movement and the anti-war movement. But mainly, he says, he has focused his life on helping generations of students learn to think for themselves. He made a specialty of teaching them how to converse in the classroom.

Claude has reached the full maturity that can come with old age. "I am alert to the small changes in my memory and in my aging body. I move slowly and sit for long stretches at a time. I wonder if this is the last time

I will see that tree in bloom or see my grandson. I feel I am returning now to what I have always been, my essential self with no need to do anything." He has accepted his aging and his disabilities with calmness and grace.

He is also aware of his own approaching death. He has spent time designing his memorial service, so it will be just as he wants it with just the right music. Death is just one more phase of development for him, not to be feared or avoided, and accepted when it is the right time. In the meantime, he is truly enjoying this last phase. For him it is a time of inner peace and reflection, a time to savor the sense of completion.

Not many eightysomethings reach this very last phase of old age where they enjoy a sense of completion. Some of us are doing things and staying busy right up to the very end. And that can be good, too. Claude shows that there is another way to be old that is in the realm of the possible. He has had the wonderful and quite rare opportunity to experience all the stages of life development and, arriving at the last stage, to be a person contented and fulfilled.

Claude's survivor skills are primarily psychological. He has let go of striving, of the need to accomplish more. He has accepted he is old, and that means he can just relax and be himself. No need to do anything more. Miguel, Jackie, Denny, and Mazelle have all let go of many aspects of their former lives in order to be where they are today. All of them are poor. None of them work anymore, and none of them (except Denny, maybe) has a role in society with influence or power. All have adapted to many losses of their physical capabilities.

To have adapted to so many losses and to be living quite happily is truly heroic. We need to learn to see the eightysomething heroes in our midst.

CONVERSATION STARTERS

- Why do you think you have survived into your eighties?
- Are you living with less? Less income, less energy? How do you manage?
- What adaptations have you made to physical disabilities and what has that been like for you?
- How have you grieved the losses of family and friends you have experienced?
- Have you gone through all the stages of grief in your eighties?

TIPS FOR FAMILIES

- Don't worry if your eightysomething is far less active than in previous years.
- If your eightysomething complains, remember that just listening to them can be healing. They may not need you to fix it.
- If your family member is more isolated than they would like to be, do some joint problem-solving. But check with them first.
- Eightysomethings fear losing their independence, but socializing and safety are important, too. If you observe they are having difficulties, be ready to step in.

CHAPTER 14

HOW THEIR KIDS SEE THEM

The children of eightysomethings live in a different world than their parents. In this chapter we will hear stories about five eightysomething parents from the perspective of the younger generation. Each parent was facing a new challenge or a change in their life situation. In families where there are number of grown kids trying to handle an evolving situation with their aging parent, it can be a recipe for conflict, confusion, and logjams.

For Martin, fifty-eight, the upset in the family equilibrium came with the arrival of a new girlfriend, Thales, into his dad's life. His dad, who was eighty-seven and living in a nursing home, had apparently known Thales twenty years previous. Thales, sixty-one, was just back in Boston after a year working overseas. She began visiting Martin's dad every day and staying for many hours. In Martin's case, he and his sister, Jo, saw Thales as a problem right from the start. She was bossy and brassy—barking orders about their dad's care to the nurses. They were annoyed at her presumption.

Soon Martin and Jo had many questions about Thales's motives. Was she trying to trick their dad into marriage, so she could get his money and his house? Had she already received big gifts from him? Martin was heavily in debt and was counting on his inheritance to get his finances squared away, and Jo needed money for her kids' college tuitions.

Martin and Jo agreed that Thales's long visits were too much for their dad and were not good for his health. They informed Thales and the nursing staff that Thales could visit only three times a week and only for an hour. Their dad said he enjoyed Thales's visits and the nurses paid no attention to their request. Thales kept visiting as usual.

"We thought we should protect our gullible dad from this wicked woman," explained Martin. As their dad began to fail, Martin became obsessed with the idea that there would be some nasty surprise for them when their dad's will was read. He and Jo considered going to their dad's lawyer to tell him about their concerns. When his dad did die a few months later, Martin was happily surprised that Thales was not even mentioned in the will. It was a bit of an anti-climax.

In this case, it seems Martin's reaction to the girlfriend was based more on fear than facts. It was mostly about money. This is a quite common scenario and sometimes the threat is real. But there are other factors at play. Primitive feelings are stirred up when grown kids see a parent with a new romantic attachment. Some of them feel it would be disloyal to their other parent, even though dead, to welcome the new relationship. Others feel upset to be displaced in theirs parent's affections. Since many of these feelings are unconscious, they are not easy to manage.

In Francene's story about her mother-in law, Rita, eighty-six, the disruptive event was Rita's serious heart condition. At this point, Anna, Rita's oldest daughter, decided it was time for her mother to move out of her house. She set up a conference call with her two brothers and her sister, Julia, to decide on a course of action. Francene, since she was a daughter-in-law, was not invited.

The phone call was noisy and long. The four siblings, according to Francene, are all "argumentative and stubborn." They did agree it was time for Rita to move and that her house should be sold. But they couldn't agree on where she should live. Since Anna worked at an insurance company with a specialty in retirement plans, she believed she was the expert and should manage Rita's move to assisted living. When they checked with Rita, she didn't want to go to assisted living; she wanted to live with Anna. Anna said, "Absolutely not."

Then Julia, the other sister, said Rita could live with her with one condition. The other three kids would have to put up money to renovate her house to make it suitable for Rita. That looked like it might work, and they decided to run with that idea. The brothers just wanted to have nothing more to do with their mom's move.

But then the quibbling began. About money. How much was reasonable for the renovations? Francene's husband claimed Julia was asking for way too much money for the renovation and refused to go further with that plan. Francene tried to smooth things over but ended up fighting with Julia. Julia said Francene and her husband had all but stolen money from her by nixing the renovation plan. Francene told me, "I couldn't believe Julia was such a bully." Rita announced she wanted to go to Anna's, not Julia's, anyhow. Anna said, "Not possible," again. Finally, Rita agreed to go to live with her sister in New York.

After two years of truce in the family warfare, Anna zoomed in again and announced that Rita must move immediately out of her sister's house. The house, she claimed, was toxic from mold and it was making Rita sick. This time Anna convinced Rita to go to an assisted living facility. The only problem was that Rita was so ultra-frugal that she picked the cheapest assisted living facility in the state. Rita found it boring and uncomfortable. After a year, Rita announced she was leaving the place. "I am going home," she said definitively. And so she did, moving back to her old house that had been rented for three years. Now, Francene told me, the kids are insisting that Rita get someone to live in the house with her. Rita, meanwhile, is sending them emails saying, "Why haven't I heard from any of you? My family takes care of their family." The story goes on and on.

This vignette illustrates how difficult it is for a family with a number of non-local adult children to sensibly manage the situation when an eightysomething needs to move. Their story is unique but the themes are typical. Here we have two sisters vying for control of their mother and the process, and two sons backing away. The difference in the behavior of the males and females is typical. None of the kids included Rita in the decision-making process. And they never develop a way to make decisions among themselves and come to closure. Finally, of course, Rita does think for herself, but only after years of trial and error and family quarrels.

There are other themes here, too. First, eightysomethings are sometimes treated like unwanted goods, like the proverbial fruitcake at Christmastime that is passed from house to house. And secondly, there are differences in attitudes between the generations about where an old person should live. Rita wants to live with family like in the old days. The kids' lives are, for the most part, too busy for that.

Traditionally, most elderly people in the United States did move in with a child when they were no longer able to live independently. In 1940, 60 percent of elders lived with one of their children. By 1980 the percentage had declined to 12 percent. This was because more of them were financially able to live independently and chose not to live with a child. By 2014, the percentage of those over eighty-five who were living with a grown child had begun to get larger, and it is now at 24 percent. This reversal is apparently a result of uncertain economic times since the Great Recession. Once again the multigenerational household is becoming more common as more elders move in with their kids and more young kids return home to live with their parents.[1]

Unlike Rita's kids, Tracey, when she moved her mother from out of state to a senior apartment near her, paid attention to her mother's preferences every step of the way. Her story, however, echoes many of the same themes. There are kids at odds with each other, mom as a bit of a pawn, and a daughter trying to make it go well.

Tracey's mom, a widow of seventeen years, was living in rural Connecticut near her stepson, Garth, and doing fine until she wasn't. She lost thirty pounds in a couple of months and began to experience more memory loss and back pain. Garth announced it was too much pressure for his wife to care for his stepmom. Tracey quickly agreed that she would help their mom move to be near her. But Garth and his wife were furious at Tracey. To this day, two years later, Tracey isn't sure exactly why—all they would say was that she wasn't grateful for what they had done for her mom for years. Garth and Tracey rarely speak nowadays.

Tracey said, "As we planned mom's move, I tried to put myself in her shoes. We went to fourteen different places before selecting the senior apartment. Mom wouldn't admit she couldn't take care of herself. So she chose a senior apartment that didn't provide many services. Yet she was adamant that it was the right place."

In some ways the move has been a success. Her mother likes the food and gained back the weight she had lost. Worried about her mom's memory, Tracey took her to be checked out. The doctor confirmed that there was memory loss, although he ruled out Alzheimer's. In the past, she and her mother used to bicker and her mom had always been highly critical of her. "She is now appreciative of everything I do," Tracy said. "I talk with her on the phone every morning and take her out once a week."

But there are challenges. Her mom stays in her room all the time and doesn't go to any of the classes or activities. She sits with others at meals but she doesn't say much, and she hasn't made any friends. She keeps saying she wishes she were in her own home.

It is hard for Tracey to see her mom, who used to be so creative and organized, be so apathetic: "I just feel so sad and I wish that she were still able to be my mother. I think she is waiting to die. But then she has been thinking and talking about dying all my life."

Tracey may have made the common mistake of waiting too long to bring her mother to the senior apartment. Since Alzheimer's was ruled out, Tracey underestimated the degree of her mother's dementia and how much her mother's capacity has diminished. It is quite possible, though, that her mother is depressed, and, with the right medications, she might be much happier and more outgoing.

Nadia, fifty-eight, and her sister and brother have a happier tale to tell. None of them live closer than a couple of hours from their mom, eighty-two, who lives in a retirement facility in a New York suburb. Nadia sees her mom about six or seven times a year. Nadia told me that she and her siblings have developed ways of caring for their mom that work for them.

The three siblings have two conference calls on Thursdays. At the first one, the three of them talk among themselves to learn if there are any new issues with their mom. Then they call their mom and have a family call, touching base and connecting. They have made these weekly conference calls for the last four years.

Besides the phone calls, each sibling has taken on a particular role with their mom. Nadia is the emotional leader, skilled at sensing how she is feeling, what she is worrying about, and in being empathic. She also lines up extra help when her mom needs that, like when she returns from a stay in the hospital. Her sister helps mom with paperwork and taxes, and her brother with the deep voice plays the role of patriarch. He can get mom to call the doctor or do something the kids think she should do, just by requesting it.

Nadia talks with mom every day, not just for the joint Thursday call. They also have an annual all girls weekend with their mom. Nadia noticed this past year that mom had slowed down. Nadia said, "I don't need her to be who she was."

Nadia and her siblings have created structures that keep them all connected and informed about how their mother is doing. Their three-way call allows for them to set an agenda for the later call with their mom and then to present a united front. Eightysomethings hate to see conflict among their adult children. It can be a kindness not to burden them with the particulars when there are differences and quarreling.

Charlie's story has yet another twist on relations between eightysomething parents and their children. Both Charlie, fifty, and his older brother

Fritz, fifty-three, were adopted. Fritz was a problem from the time he was a teenager. He saw a number of psychiatrists and therapists but has never been able to hold a real job. Charlie feels his parents have always been preoccupied with Fritz. Now that his parents are in their eighties, that has not changed. The parents have bought a house for Fritz near them and see Fritz every day. "They are consumed by my brother, looking after him," Charlie observed.

Charlie runs a real estate business and has four kids, one from his first marriage and three from his second marriage. Charlie worries that he should do more for his parents, but they make that very hard. And he seems angry at them at the same time. He told me his dad drinks too much, and only talks about business with him. They rarely get beyond rental properties in their conversations. Charlie would like his parents to know his kids better. But although Charlie and his wife often invite them to visit, they rarely come. They tell him they are uncomfortable being far from Fritz. As for Charlie's relationship with Fritz, they see each other even less often. "We never talk. I don't see that changing."

Charlie persists in trying to get his parents' attention. Of course, where there is a troubled child, even a fifty-three-year-old troubled child, it is common for parents to continue to focus on their wounded one. And the healthier grown children, like Charlie, can continue to be neglected. And to feel neglected. But what is interesting is how hard Charlie is trying year after year to have a closer relationship with his parents and to connect them to his kids.

What, then, is to be learned from our exploration of the kids' sides of the stories? First, ties to parents are among the deepest attachment of our lives. Parents are always hugely important in forming who we have become. And these strong feelings remain strong throughout one's whole life. When parents are old, frail, and approaching death, the feelings of adult children about what is happening to them become even more intense and sometimes overwhelming. As we have seen, the children, driven by these intense feelings, can have strong and conflicting opinions about what to do.

When an eightysomething parent experiences a sudden, but not totally unexpected crisis, there is often a need for quick decisions. But what happens? The adult children regress. Instead of acting like mature adults, the old sibling patterns of childhood get reactivated. The kids lose their tempers and fight the way they used to as kids. These patterns are deeply ingrained and hard to change. With the pressure to do something quickly, it is no wonder it so hard to keep cool and act wisely.

Some eightysomethings have no adult children to fall back on. In many cases other family members—nieces, nephews, cousins, or godchildren—will step up and take on a major role in their care. But there are some eightysomethings, so called "elder orphans" who are without any family to care for them despite the large number of their cohort who had children, 83 percent.[2] According to an article in *Current Gerontology and Geriatrics Research,* "It is always high risk to be an eightysomething, totally unconnected to family and friends. It is a far worse situation than having children who lose their cool. Isolation is never good for well-being, and it negatively affects health and life expectancy."[3]

As eightysomethings live longer, stay healthier, and live more active lives than earlier generations, the role of their adult children is evolving, too. What has not changed is that today's adult children are still the key players as their aging parents decline. The kids need to understand that what they do to help and to care will shift dramatically as their parent evolves along the continuum of independence to dependence.

Once kids understand where their parent is on this continuum, it is easier to adjust how often they intervene and how much control they exert as their parent changes. There can be too much control from the kids, as in Rita's case, and too little, as in Tracey's case. Adult kids need to be aware that their parents can't go on being independent forever and need to realize how helpful an early discussion before any crisis happens can be.

They must figure out together what is the preferred course of action if the parent's health takes a serious turn for the worse.

What is most important of all is that family is still what matters most to eightysomethings, and no matter what the ups and downs in their relationships with their children have been over the years, those bonds are almost unbreakable. Adult children will almost always respond to the needs of their aging parent with love.

CONVERSATION STARTERS

- When you face major decisions nowadays, how much do you depend on your children or other family member?
- Have you moved in your eighties and if so, what did you learn from that process?
- Can you speak up and tell your children when they seem not to be listening to your needs and wants?
- Have you made a plan for what to do if your situation changes suddenly?

TIPS FOR FAMILIES

- Be sure to include your eightysomething in discussions about their care as long as possible.
- Family meetings when an eightysomething is in crisis are helpful.
- Bring in an expert like a social worker if there is a stalemate or unresolvable conflict among the adult children.
- Don't wait too long to move your eightysomething parent to an appropriate setting for them.

CHAPTER 15

SPIRITUALITY

Neal is a retired clergyman who has experienced a tsunami of doubt. He lives in an assisted living facility in suburban Chicago and is struggling with advanced prostate cancer and debilitating neuropathy. The day I met with him, he arrived at our meeting place slowly pushing a walker. His transition from walker to chair is another slow process requiring time and attention. While his thin body is bent and twisted, he has a youthful look with a full head of mostly brown hair and large blue eyes. He seems to be enjoying the human comedy that is his life at eighty-one.

He has had a long and complicated spiritual journey. In high school he was helped by his pastor to win scholarships both to college and to seminary. The 1950s were a time of incredible excitement in the religious world with teachers like Paul Tillich and William Sloane Coffin igniting a younger generation of ministers. Neal describes himself in his early years as a Zen Methodist—Zen because of his interest in spiritual discipline, and Methodist because of his roots in scripture.

After a decade serving as a parish minister, Neal attended several courses on religion and psychology that inspired him to get formal clinical training and redirect his career. He spent the next few decades working at pastoral counseling centers. As the years went by, Neal found himself shedding more and more of the rigidities of formal religion. He was frustrated by some of the conservative values of his denomination and more skeptical of doctrines like the resurrection and the virgin birth. He told me that recently he had read some of his old sermons and he was horrified at how dry and intellectual they were. Now he believes that the church belongs out in the streets. He asked me if I realized that Jesus was actually a community organizer. With a wry smile, he said, "Today I have only one small doubt, and that is about whether God actually exists or not."

When Neal notices that someone in his assisted living facility seems to be searching for spiritual guidance, he will stop and talk with them. He calls the place where he is as one of honest doubting. "I try to keep doors open. I see myself as a steward of the mysteries." He talks with others who are searching and finds them something to read. He sees himself as "one beggar telling another beggar where to find food."

Whatever his changing views of doctrine, what I noticed during our interview was how fully present he was to me. Despite his significant pain and his doubts, he remains attuned to the needs of the souls of others.

Neal's practice of religion has been altered in many ways by his aging. Now, like many eightysomethings, he no longer has a formal role in any religious organization, and his physical condition limits his attendance at his church. And his life purpose has changed, too.

Viktor Frankl, an Austrian psychiatrist, who was imprisoned at the Auschwitz concentration camp during World War II, taught us about the impact of having a purpose. He observed that the very few who survived the horror and hardships of the camp were not, as he expected, the most hardy and robust people. Rather, they were people who had a purpose for living through the suffering. It might be the hope for being united with their wife or child, or it might be a piece of work they wanted to accomplish that was what kept them alive.[1]

Frankl's book teaches us the power of having a purpose. His observations are relevant to those eightysomethings at the last stage of life when they may feel unclear about their purpose. Stripped of their roles and former ways of being, they need to develop an answer to the question, "What is my purpose for still being here?" Neal has found a new purpose for living as a "steward of the mysteries" that is possible for him despite his disabilities. This informal role gives him, even with all his doubts, a new kind of ministry. Neal can be described as a religious person who has evolved into a spiritual one.

Neal's increasing doubts echo the national story in the United States that people are gradually becoming less religious. But he is different from the vast majority of eightysomethings who stay fully committed to their religious beliefs as they age.

Here is the big picture of religion in the United States today. The United States is more religious than any other developed country in the world. Even a majority of Americans without religious affiliations say they believe in God and two thirds of adults pray every day, according to the Pew Research Center US Religious Landscape Study of 2014. There are an incredibly large number of different religions and denominations with which Americans are affiliated. Here is the breakdown of the US population by major religious groups in this country.

US Population by Religion

Christian	70.6%	(Protestant, Catholic, and other)
Non-Christian	5.9%	(Jewish, Muslim, Buddhist, Hindu)
Unaffiliated	23.5%	(Atheist, Agnostic, religious "nones")[2]

Now, some clarification on the difference between religion and spirituality. The concepts of religion and spirituality are overlapping, not separate; it is a difference in emphasis.

Religious people are those who are connected to institutions and community. They are part of a system of faith and beliefs and follow certain designated behaviors, practices, and rituals. Spiritual people, on the other hand, engage in practices that are more individually focused and less formal. They may be within or outside a religious institution. Spiritual practices might include lighting candles, meditating, fasting, praying, and looking at the stars. Spirituality has been called a quest to transcend the ordinary limits of human experience.

As they age, the majority of eightysomethings are more observant than younger generations. They report that religion is their largest source of support outside the family. They volunteer at their religious organization more frequently than at any other place.

Lenore, Joan, and Gautam are three people whose stories, along with Neal's, begin to suggest the varieties of religious and spiritual experience among eightysomethings in the United States.

In contrast to Neal's ever increasing doubts, Lenore is a born-again Christian whose faith has never wavered throughout her long life. She, the youngest of seven children, grew up on a farm at the edge of a tiny town in North Dakota. Her parents, who had come from Sweden, belonged to a Lutheran church with strict rules. As a girl, Lenore worked on the farm, was active in the church, sang in the choir, and participated in the youth group.

Lenore married young and moved to another farm and another Lutheran church where she continued to work hard, teach Sunday school, and sing in the choir. She raised five kids. Then one winter, when she was about forty, the weather was so severe that for many Sundays they could not get to church. She began watching a TV evangelist who preached dramatic sermons about Jesus and the good news. One day, at home, she found herself kneeling beside the kitchen table. She heard a deep, calm, and reassuring voice telling her, "Now you don't need to be afraid of dying." And she knew she was transformed for life, almost like she was a new person, born again. For a year she was afraid to tell her husband about this experience. But many months later when she did tell him, he understood.

In 1980, terrible storms ruined all the crops on their farm and they just couldn't pay the debts that had accumulated over the years. They had to sell the farm and move to a new town. Her husband became a beekeeper and the family prospered again. But it was not easy for her, she explained; she was lonely because she was now a Swede living in a Norwegian community.

Today Lenore, whose large, plump body radiates warmth and comfort, has been living in an assisted living facility for four years. She has endured many losses. Her husband died six years ago. Her children live hours away. She has had two hip and two knee replacements. Last year she fell and damaged her right hand and can't really use that hand at all. This makes daily life difficult. "The Lord took away things so now I have more time for other things. My faith in Jesus sustains me," she said. She explained that most of the people at her facility are retired farm people. They all have problems, but they are so reserved that it is hard for them to reach out. She sees herself as an "encourager"—she greets them, listens to their problems, and tells them that the Lord loves them.

Every night she reads the Bible for an hour after dinner and prays after that. She prays in the mornings too. Only one of her kids is a churchgoer, but she keeps praying for all the others to come back to the church. "These are extreme times, I see terrible things going on all around—the kids today, they know too much." She prays for peace in Jerusalem before Jesus comes again. She is also interested in a group of untouchables in India that have been "saved" and whose faith is growing. She wishes that the number of faithful would grow more quickly.

As Lenore has aged, her faith, as always, continues to be her major coping mechanism. "It has all been so simple for me," she said. She feels that despite all the losses she has experienced, "all will be well." She has an attitude of calm acceptance, whatever life throws her way. And her life today with so few responsibilities allows her to spend even more time each day in prayer and reading the Bible. She has also, like Neal, evolved and developed a new purpose for her present life, in her case to be an "encourager" of the other residents at her facility.

Unlike Lenore, whose religious life has been lived out in the midst of people and organizations, Joan's spiritual life has always been solitary. Joan is a New Yorker who, at eighty-four, is a weaver and still takes ballet lessons three times a week. She stands tall and straight, her long gray hair hanging far down her back. Twice divorced, she lives alone now that her cat has died. She scrapes by by selling a few wall hangings each year and with some help from her second ex-husband who remains a loving friend. She said:

> I do not describe myself as religious, I am spiritual. I feel I am not separate from the all of nature—the sea, the wind, and the earth.
>
> Forty years ago, one hot July afternoon, while I was running in the city, I sought the cool darkness of a monastery chapel. I was such a mess that I had been cutting my arms and I was still ruminating about my childhood abuse by my uncle. The music of the Evensong and the simplicity of the architecture of chapel soothed me that day and I found myself unexpectedly at peace. I have continued to go the chapel for years; there is something there. Is it the Holy Spirit? I don't know, but I can work things out, wrestle with my problems. The place is not a social gathering. You can go and not talk with anybody. It allows you to be very private.
>
> Yes, I pray, and it is okay for you to ask about that. I pray in the morning and at night—for all the world, the people who are on the street, immigrants, the poor, my brother, for healing of others. But today I am afraid. I have been diagnosed with a

serious heart condition. I realize that now I, myself, am in need of healing. That is a surprise for me. I have always been so strong—not focused on me.

Joan's spiritual life has been grounded in one particular place, the monastery chapel, for forty years. As a fiercely independent introvert, she does not want to depend on anyone. But now, in this last stage of life, she is essentially in crisis. She has a serious medical condition and it looks like her lifestyle is in jeopardy. Her vulnerability makes her feel terribly unsettled. As a psychotherapist, I wonder if she will be able to reach out for help from friends, her former husband, her brother, or her old therapist. I hope she can allow herself to be dependent, to lean on others now that she is no longer strong. To be able to be dependent is one of the key tasks for all eightysomethings.

Like Joan, Gautam, eighty-nine, who lives in northern New Jersey, is not affiliated with any religious organization. His skepticism dates way back to early childhood faith. Gautam is a Hindu who was born in India in the merchant caste. His mother often went to temple and practiced many rituals and ceremonies in the home, like fasting every Tuesday. He remembers when he was eight years old telling his mother, "This is silly."

Gautam came to this country for graduate work when he was nineteen. He worked for Bethlehem Steel, and other mining companies before becoming a consultant. He has been married three times; once, he told me, to a WASP and twice to Jewish women, all of whom have died. Now he lives alone in an apartment decorated with objects from India. He is tall and sturdy, and, as he made sure to tell me, he looks as if he is in his seventies.

As far as his beliefs, Gautam believes in God. With all his skepticism, this astonished me. His God, he explained, is not like a man. It is a power that is at the center of a wheel and all spokes lead to this God. Gautam gives thanks for all that he has, for being well and alive. But that is it. He is not interested in any ritual or ceremonies. Of course, he told me, "I am not a typical Hindu if that's what you are looking for, I am more cosmopolitan and tolerant." Many Hindus in the United States, he noted, go often to temple and listen to gurus on the radio. Gautam thinks many of these spiritual teachers are "rogues."

He explained how in the Hindu culture, old people are venerated. Gautam remembers how whenever he saw one of his grandparents he would greet them by touching their foot as an act of respect. They, in turn, would give him a blessing. It was a mutual exchange demonstrating their esteem for each other. His children are American, so they have no concept of veneration, he said a bit sadly. And now, regrettably, the elderly Hindus in his suburban town are facing the last stage of life as individuals, each on their own, not as a community. What is new, now, is that he realizes the need for connection to other Hindus as he is in the last stage of life. It makes sense to face death in the company of others, in community.

Like Neal, my own religious life been one of change rather than continuity. I come from a long line of Calvinist preachers and teachers. But by the time I was born, any religious fervor had long since been extinguished. We were a rational family more than a religious or spiritual one. In my twenties, that changed for me. My husband and I participated in a study group of six couples that met with our minister every other Sunday night for five years. We laughed, cried, shared our deepest concerns, sometimes read the Bible, and learned about Carl Jung. I experienced the amazing power of a loving group to bring about personal transformation. Religion and psychology were interconnected. We all became more courageous, more confident, and more loving. When John took a job in another state, we had to leave that group that was so important to me. After years of abortive attempts to find a spiritual home, I found Unitarian Universalism. I was attracted to the sense of community and the commitment to social justice.

And as so often happens nowadays, my children have brought more diversity and change to our family. One daughter-in-law is Jewish. Next week I will attend the Bat Mitzvah of my granddaughter, Aliya. Two other daughters-in-law were brought up Catholic. One of them is now Presbyterian, but her daughter refused to be confirmed this year. She told the minister she thought she might be Unitarian like her grandmother.

For most people, whatever their religion, it changes significantly as they age into their eighties. The hustle and bustle of church, of organized religious life, does not usually match their changing needs and lessening stamina. The task as always, is to be at a place on the spiritual pathway that is just right for their needs at present moment. Not to retreat from the world too soon. Not to hold on to old ways too long. In her book *Who Am I . . . Now That I'm Not Who I Was?* Connie Goldman, formerly on the staff at NPR, put it this way, "The journey in between who I once was and who I am now becoming is where the dance of life really takes place."[3] Good counsel, we can keep evolving no matter how old we are.

CONVERSATION STARTERS

- Has your practice of religion shifted now that you are in your eighties?
- How have your beliefs shifted over the years?
- Do you find yourself more interested in spiritual matters and the inner life in your eighties? How so?
- How have you redefined your purpose now that you are eighty?

TIPS FOR FAMILIES

- Is your eightysomething attending religious services? If not, ask if they would like to.

- See if they would like to talk about how their beliefs have evolved as they have aged.
- Ask about what religious or spiritual beliefs have guided them their whole life.
- Inquire if they have a spiritual practice that that means a lot to them now that they are an eightysomething.

CHAPTER 16

APPROACHING DEATH

Most people of every age push away thoughts of death. Eightysomethings are no exception. Arnold Toynbee, a British philosopher of history, once said that death was un-American. He was right because, for most of us, our prevailing attitude toward death is denial. Kate Sweeney, an award-winning writer about death, said, "Americans are so obsessed with youth and triumphing over every challenge they face that they become afraid of aging and death, often seen as life's ultimate defeat."[1] Living in a culture where people are trying to look and act young makes bringing up the subject of death practically taboo.

In the past, babies, children, and adults of all ages died at far higher rates than today. So, everyone grew up experiencing many people around them dying. In the last fifty years, modern medicine has lowered the death rate and increased longevity dramatically. Death is not so familiar now and it is often thought of as something that comes with old age. Many people today tend to think about death as a problem that can be solved by medical advancements. And so they focus their attention on breakthrough cures that address the major causes of death. They ignore death's inevitability.

Since denial of death is so pervasive in the United States, it can be surprising to learn that Buddhist monks in Thailand often contemplate photos of corpses. It is said that the Buddha himself often meditated while looking at dead bodies. He recommended the practice, believing that thinking about death can lead to living a better life. The Romans had the same idea with their saying, *momento mori*—remember you are going to die—implying, do this so you can live well. Olivia Hoblitzelle, who wrote *Aging with Wisdom,* came up with a mantra for her own aging: Contemplate death. Be grateful and be joyful.[2]

At my retirement community, made up of mostly eightysomethings, death is a frequent visitor. So despite the denial of its presence, death takes on an aspect of the everyday and ordinary. The first thing I do each day when I go to the lobby is to walk over to the case where death announcements are displayed. *Good, no one has died overnight.*

Years ago, rumor has it, they used to place a white rose in a vase beside the death announcements. By the time I arrived, however, they had replaced real roses with a picture of a rose on a paper announcement. The budget was tight in those years, but still, it seemed unnecessarily frugal. When they finally installed a new bronze and glass case with dignified announcements accompanied by real roses, there was universal approval. Gravitas is needed when it comes to death.

Although denial of death is typical of eightysomethings like everyone else, it is also obvious that death is drawing closer. There are all sorts of variations on how eightysomethings deal with their approaching death given these two sets of facts side by side. I'll start with the example of Gene, who is an extreme denier.

Gene told me with just a suggestion of sarcasm in his voice, "I just don't believe that I am going to die. It is always the other guy. I just don't think about it." Gene is a busy man living in New York. He has had a couple of careers and a couple of wives. He was a lawyer and then was in business until his eighties. At eighty-four, he is still "uncommonly healthy," playing tennis and senior softball and going out to movies and concerts about three times a week. He does have a bit of arthritis and admits it takes longer for wounds to heal. "I guess I am a freak—I can run around and play ball. I am a free spirit. Most other people seem so goal-oriented, but I am just enjoying the journey. And I just keep moving."

I believe Gene when he says he doesn't think he will die. While he knows that is not possible, he also knows he *is* different from most people his age. His good health allows him to keep rowing merrily, merrily down the stream. He can stay in denial far longer than most of his peers whose lists of health issues are far longer than his. But is that the best way to live?

This extreme denial has its downsides as well as its upsides. He may have neglected to make a will and may have given no thought about his own hopes for how he would want care at the end of life. Only one in five people have communicated their wishes for their end of life care and their dying to their family.[3] This can mean a lot of confusion when there is a crisis.

Unlike Gene, Maureen, eighty-two, who is a retired nurse, told me in a matter-of-fact kind of way that she is quite prepared to die. "I've talked with my husband and we've made plans. We don't want to be cremated. We have wills, health proxies, and have talked about our funerals. But, having done all that, that's it, we're done. We have never had another conversation about dying." She feels she should be doing something more but can't figure out exactly what that is.

Maureen and her husband have taken care of business in terms of preparing for dying. In that sense she is way ahead of most people in the United States who often die without wills or health proxies. But now that a few basics are covered, she and her husband, just like Gene, avoid the topic. She has replaced denial with avoidance. She is right, it would be better if she and her husband could have some conversations about what they each want at the end of their life. What means the most to them in terms of their last weeks and months? How can they be there for each other at the end? What if they can't talk or speak and have major cognitive decline?

Cassy, eighty-seven, is a person who is ready to die. (You met her in chapter 2, the joyful and stoic woman with so many health issues.) In her case, it was a near-death experience more than fifty years ago during the birth of her son that gave her peace of mind about dying: "Something went wrong during the birth. I could hear the doctors and nurses scrambling to do something. Then it was quiet and I was suddenly bathed in a golden light. I did not want to come back. I heard a voice saying, 'Pay attention, it matters.' And I slowly and reluctantly came back from the other side."

This experience changed Cassy. "I realized that all I have to do is to pay attention to living; I did not need to worry about dying. What it meant to me was to be open to any situation. Listen, and don't close up or judge what someone else should do. And the peace of that golden light has been with me ever since. I am ready to go. Sooner is fine. But I do want to be present for the finale."

Losing her friends has not been easy for Cassy. Four of her five closest friends have died in the last two years. She said, "I just can't move on, I need time to think about what I have lost. So I take silent retreats, with just me, to think about what I lost with the death of each one." About six months after our interview, I learned that Cassy died. I hope she was present, the way she wanted, for the finale.

Several other people I interviewed had near-death experiences. One eightysomething man, during heart surgery twenty years earlier, had become aware that he had died. He remembered that he felt peaceful on the other side. But then, he came back. And like Cassy, the impact has been that he is no longer afraid of dying. In addition, he feels sure that there is some kind of afterlife.

My own attitude toward dying is less about denial and more about anxiety. Death in my family comes suddenly. My father went out to shovel snow for a few minutes and when he returned to the house, my mother had died. It was totally unexpected and out of the blue. She was sixty-five. My father died when he was seventy-one, as he was chatting away at dinner on a cruise. Since I turned sixty-five, it occurs to me quite often that this day might be the day I die. Like my parents, out of the blue. I was surprised to discover from my interviews that not many people have thoughts like that.

Judith's story was different from most others, too. No denial for her, as she has made death her life's work. A licensed psychologist, now eighty-four, living in northern California, Judith looked overwhelmed the day I met up with her—make-up slightly askew and dyed blonde hair every which way. She informed me, "I am still at it, working for better laws. It is terrible that there is still so much needless suffering as people reach the end of life."

According to Judith, only a few states, like Oregon, have laws that make sense and allow for death with dignity. As far back as 1987, Judith was active in the Hemlock Society, an organization that advocated for assisted suicide. For years, she traveled around the world to spread the word. When the Society folded in 2003, she turned her efforts to the Final Exit Network that provides mentors to those seeking to die at a moment of their own choosing.

Today, Judith admitted she just doesn't have the energy to do much work with any organization. Her apartment is a mess, and she can't seem to get organized to clean up the clutter. And what is new for her, she is no longer thinking much about dying. How interesting.

Since there is usually resistance to talking about death, especially among people who are actually approaching death, I was intrigued when a woman at my retirement community told me she was organizing a whole series of events called "Let's Talk about Death." It would include several films and presentations on palliative care and hospice, green burials, and maintaining control at the end of life.

It would also include a death café, a facilitated event where people sit at tables, sip tea and eat cake, and most importantly, talk about death. There is no formal agenda, just a facilitator to keep time and guide a discussion at the end. It is based on the premise that, although most people do avoid conversations about death, they have thoughts and concerns about death that go unexpressed. And a number of people have a yearning to talk with others about these thoughts. The assumption is that by talking about death they will begin to face the reality of it. This, in turn, may enable them to live fuller, more joyful lives. Death cafés have been held all over the world and the concept is something of a global movement now.

But talking about death *is* a sensitive a topic for eightysomethings. Some at our retirement community were upset when it was announced that the speaker about green burials was planning to bring several biodegradable caskets to our lecture hall. (The idea was quashed.) Other people were upset just by the idea of a death café—to them it seemed disrespectful and even sacrilegious. They wouldn't attend. We wondered if anyone would come.

Despite the worry ahead of time, at the actual death café there was spirited conversation at all four tables. At the end, people shared what it had meant to them. Among the comments were: "I really appreciated the chance to talk about my father's death." "It was so good, because I can't talk like this with my wife." "It was nice to have a serious conversation, I couldn't imagine that people would open up like we did." "When can we do this again?"

Using *Five Wishes* as a guide is another way to have a conversation about the end of life and to plan for it. It meets legal requirements in forty-two states and is useful in all. More than eighteen million copies of *Five Wishes* have been distributed by more than thirty-five thousand organizations.

A person's responses to each of the wishes lets their family and doctors know about what kind of experience and care they want at the end of their life. It is helpful in that it speaks to medical, personal, emotional, and spiritual needs. The results of a conversation can end up as a living will, a document that will be helpful when that last stage is reached. The Five Wishes are:

1. Who you want to make health care decisions for you when you can't make them.
2. What kind of medical treatment you want or don't want.
3. How comfortable you want to be.
4. How you want people to treat you.
5. What you want your loved ones to know.

Another useful tool is the Conversation Project, which provides a starter kit for families to begin talking about death and wishes for end-of-life care for a family member who may be dying. Most families avoid having these conversations and keep putting them off. The Conversation Project's guide has helped many families come to a shared understanding of what matters most to those approaching the last stage of life.

Hospice care is a relatively new option for care, now available in many parts of the country, that is changing how we treat the dying. The purpose of hospice is to bring dignity, quality of life, and comfort to those near the end of their life, rather than focusing on curing them. Hospice sees the dying as multifaceted people, far more than just people with serious medical problems. Hospice staff attend to the emotional and spiritual needs of the entire family, not just the dying.

In most cases, hospice provides care right in the home, although at times people are at a hospital or a nursing home. Hospice is free for those on Medicare and is usually covered for most people on Medicaid and by most insurance plans. Preparation can make things go more smoothly for everyone. Of course, the reality is you can have all documents and conversations ahead of time and things can still go wrong. EMTs do not get the message. Families and doctors can't face carrying out the wishes. The laws in many states can make it difficult. But having a plan, and having the right documents, can prevent untold misery.

In our fifties, John and I talked about how we wanted to die. It happened because of Arthur, an older man who was our acquaintance. When

Arthur was dying, he retreated to his attic. He didn't tell anybody he had cancer—he couldn't even say the word, and he didn't want any visitors to see him as he declined. John and I agreed this was not how we wanted to be. We hoped to be more open and not so alone.

Many years later, as John was dying, we did bring in family and friends to be there, along with me, to see him on his way out. He was surrounded by those who loved him, those who wanted to come: his four sons and their wives, some of the grandchildren, the old friends with whom we had gathered for dinners for twenty years, and new friends from the retirement community.

What also helped during John's departing days was a small group of singers from our church who came eight or nine times to sing at his bedside. He would hum along at times, sleep sometimes, and have an expression of pure joy on his face at other times. These songs for the dying were an amazing gift to both of us.

Then it helped that each morning of John's last week, the chaplain at our retirement community came to my apartment and said prayers for John and me and one or two or three of my non-believing sons who were there. Those prayers were soothing and uplifting. They provided a context of meaning to John's death. They gave us a sense that John's dying and our family were part of a much larger tradition and community that was holding us safely, believers and non-believers, in our sorrow.

Because people in their eighties know they are approaching death, when they do move beyond avoidance and denial of death, they often surprisingly suddenly experience unexpected happiness. They can take pleasure in the present moment and what remains, rather than thinking about all that has been lost. They are finally able to feel at peace and ready to welcome death whenever it comes.

CONVERSATION STARTERS

- Have you taken care of the basic preparations for dying including a will and a healthcare proxy?
- What have you decided about what you want done with your body when you die, what kind of service you want, and where you want to be buried? And have you written this down and told your family?
- Have you used *Five Wishes* to communicate to your family about what kind of care you want for yourself at the end of life?
- What is your plan if your condition suddenly takes a turn for the worst? Where do you want to be?

TIPS FOR FAMILIES

- Check in with your eightysomething about where they stand in terms of practical documents preparing for their death. Help them with the process of getting these done if they have not done them already.
- Go through the *Five Wishes* with your eightysomething. It may take several conversations. Be sure to put into a document what their wishes are.
- Prepare for your own death now by taking care of the practical matters of a will, and other advance directives.
- When a family member is dying, remember, just being there with them in person is the greatest gift.

CHAPTER 17

UNEXPECTEDLY HAPPY

I love being in my eighties," said Patty, "Just being alive is special. None of my family lived past seventy, so I never expected to be here now." Patty, eighty-two, is a tall, lanky woman wearing khaki pants and a flannel shirt. She has lived alone since her husband left her more than twenty-five years ago. She added, "And I have learned to like it, living alone. I love spring and gardening. I grow vegetables and flowers. Each day I make a list of what I want to do. Get the beans started. Go shopping. Go to church. But if I don't get things done it's okay. No pressure to get things done. My life is all easy and pleasant."

"That's not to say I haven't been through a lot in my life," Patty acknowledged, and she went on to explain that her daughter was murdered twenty years ago. The past year her daughter-in-law died, and her son is miserable being alone. She has no grandkids. She has financial problems. Her health is pretty good except she passed out a couple of times recently and had to go to the emergency room. It's her heart. Even with all this, Patty rated her level of happiness as *very happy*, a nine on a scale of one to ten.

Patty demonstrates that, for some people in their eighties, being happy does not depend on having avoided setbacks, failures, and tragedies. It is often unexpected, though. In Patty's case, her happiness seemed related to the freedom and calm in her day-to-day life. And the high level of happiness that so many eightysomethings feel was one of my major findings. And, also, one of the surprises.

A groundbreaking research study conducted by Judith Rodin and Ellen

Langer back in the 1970s shed more light on the factors undergirding Patty's happiness. Rodin and Langer looked at two similar groups of elderly residents in two wings of a large nursing home. Before the study, the groups had been evaluated as having equivalent levels of health. During the months of the study, those in the experimental group were given choices about many aspects of their daily life and were encouraged to express their preferences. For example, they were asked to decide when to see movies and where they wished to see their visitors. Each of them was given a plant to care for. In the control group, nursing staff made all the decisions about the schedule and took care of the plants in each room.

Rodin and Langer expected that after several months of the study, the experimental group, with more options and more choices, would express more satisfaction and contentedness than those in the control group. And they did. They were also judged to be more alert and active than the control group. Rodin and Langer believed this showed that older people were more capable than staff or families realized. They had learned to be helpless when they were not given choices or responsibilities. Rodin and Langer saw the results of their study as clearly demonstrating this idea of learned helplessness. The experimental group's health had also shown significant improvement after the study, while those in the control group had no change.

But then came a surprising finding. The results of the study also showed a significant difference between the number of people who had died in the two groups. In the control group, 30 percent of them had died during the study compared to only 15 percent in the experimental group. This stunning experiment has been replicated many times, and the findings hold up. More choices, more decision-making possibilities, and more responsibility raise the level of happiness in older people. These things also keep them healthier. And most importantly, they keep them alive.[1]

So back to Patty. What makes her happy is that she has much control over her life. She can do what she wants day by day. And she not only has a plant to care for, she has a whole garden to tend.

Connie, like Patty, told me she is "very happy." She is the woman who was a caretaker of her husband for ten years whom you read about in chapter 8. She has pure white hair, blue eyes, and cheeks bright pink with powder. She was smiling as I began our second interview. Her smile never left her face.

I asked about her life in her still new apartment. She started with how cozy it is. She loves being there. She said her recliner chair is her home; everything she needs is within reach—glasses, phone, paper and pencil, calendar, date book, books, and walker. She always has a fire burning in the gas fireplace. She glowed as she told me that the day before she was able to resume swimming after a four-week break while she was recovering from a bout of bronchitis. "You can't believe how wonderful it is. It is pure joy to just lie there in the water, floating. It is so peaceful. All my worries fly away," she said.

Our conversation turned to a less joyful topic, her daughter, Sabina. She explained how Sabina has been difficult her whole life. She didn't finish high school and has rarely had a job. Now at fifty, she is a divorced mom who needs to find work. Meanwhile Connie has been giving her money.

Connie said, "Some days Sabina is loving and helpful to me, but last week she came here and yelled at me. She said that I am a controlling bitch and what a horrible mother I have been. I cried for a whole day." Connie's sons told her not to listen to Sabina, that she is a nut case.

She continued, "I am okay. I am happy when I am not seeing Sabina and worrying about her problems." Connie believes that Sabina needs some medication. And Connie is upset that her sons are mad at her because she has been supporting Sabina. "I will keep seeing her and giving her money because she is my daughter."

From my point of view as a psychotherapist, Sabina has serious mental health issues. She needs to see a doctor, preferably a psychiatrist, who could prescribe some medication for her that will help her mood swings.

Connie said, "Another thing that makes me unhappy is the news. So I don't look at TV because there is nothing good there. Of course, I have so much to be grateful for. I have met so many lovely friends here and there are good classes and the large pool. When I stay in my apartment for a whole day, I am happy then, too, just being by myself."

Connie has developed an ability to block out from her awareness the negative aspects of her life—her worries about her daughter and the larger world—so that much of the time she can feel happy and calm. It's almost a daily act of willpower to chase away the darkness.

Ethan, unlike Patty and Connie, is an example of an eightysomething who is unhappy. His opening remark to me was, "Life is a fatal disease." He is a large man with a full head of brown-gray hair and a slightly disheveled look. Retired for years, Ethan was a physicist who worked at a company that conducted research for the government. Now eighty-two, he is still on his computer every day, all day, although he is no longer able to work through difficult problems: "Yet, I like tackling them even if I am not going to succeed." He elaborated in a mournful voice, "I make so many mistakes and at the end of a week, I just haven't progressed. I get so damn frustrated."

What else does he do? He reported he doesn't play video games but he does exercise and take walks. "I am less strong than I was when I was younger, have less energy. Climbing stairs is starting to be difficult." He goes to church almost every week. He rates his happiness level as a five, well below the average of those I interviewed.

Ethan is still striving to achieve and has not made his peace with his declining mental prowess, or his aging for that matter. He is comparing himself today to himself in his prime and this comparison makes him unhappy day after day. His pattern of working is so much a part of him and he hasn't been able to modify his lifestyle. Successful aging requires accepting change and focusing on what remains.

Clive is another happy eightysomething. Like Patty and Connie, he has family problems, but he has also had some good luck. A former electrical engineer and flight test engineer, he lives in Seattle.

He told me:

Here I am at eighty-one taking care of both my mother who is ninety-nine and also my wife. My wife is high strung and high maintenance. I have been the steady hand, doing everything in the home for decades. But when anything goes wrong, she blames me. She resents the time I spend with my mother. It has been rough for fifty-three years.

I also worry about my grandson, who is having problems at school. I think his parents are far too permissive. I was brought up by my conservative grandparents, who had old-fashioned ideas. So I have had no inclination for drugs or drink. They taught me that your body is your temple, so don't mistreat it.

I did win one million dollars from the state lottery some years ago. How did it change me? Well, it made life a little easier so I could put some money aside. Actually nothing changed. I still worked and life went on as usual. I felt I had to tell the bishop about the lottery. Then, having spilled the beans, I felt obligated to make a huge gift to the church.

I have no close friends, but go places with my two sons, football games, concerts. I like jazz and blues. I used to play piano and trombone. I belong to the AME Zion church and go most weeks. I used to sing in the choir but I am taking a break. I go to the senior citizen center for exercise class three times a week.

Clive rates his current level of happiness as an eight. "I am a history buff, and, as a black man, particularly interested in the Tuskegee Airmen," he said. The Tuskegee Airman were the nine hundred African American men trained by the Army Air Corps in World War II as pilots, navigators, and bombardiers. Clive has gone to many of their reunions and is sad that their number is dwindling away.

Clive was a lucky man to win a million dollars in a state lottery. Much as we would imagine it might have made for a better life, he reported that it didn't change anything.

A recent report about a classic study that compared the happiness of paraplegics and winners of a lottery—helps us understand why winning the lottery didn't change anything for Clive. The findings of the study were that paraplegics experienced more pleasure in their day-to-day activities than winners of the Illinois state lottery. The analysis of why this was true is that the burst of joy that comes with winning a lottery wears off quickly. The lives of the winners soon return to the way they were before their windfall. Paraplegics, similarly, apparently over time, adapt to their condition. Most paraplegics were not born that way; at some point in time they went through a traumatic accident. Since then, they evaluate the ups and downs of their daily life within the confines of their new situation. It is the day to day that makes for happiness.[2]

This is similar to how eightysomethings experience their lives. They adapt over time to their conditions and their individual limitations become taken for granted. It is usually the ups and downs within those limits that create the sense of joy or misery. For example, when Connie's bronchitis was gone, she was happy. When she thinks about her daughter, she is unhappy. And when people, such as Ethan, continue to hold themselves to the standard of their selves of yesteryears, they feel dissatisfied.

So, Clive reported his level of happiness was not raised by winning the lottery, and it apparently has not been lowered by his relationship with his demanding wife and his mother. He has got to be one of the only eightysomethings in the country who is caring for his mother. We have seen from the Rodin and Langer study that having responsibilities can increase happiness. For Clive this means that caring for both his mother and his wife probably contributes to his happiness. Clive rated his happiness as an eight, very happy. He likes spending time with his mother despite the fact that his wife resents it.

Laura Carstensen, a professor of psychology at Stanford University and founder of the Stanford Center for Longevity, helps us understand why older people generally report higher levels of happiness than any other age group—more than younger people or middle-aged people. She wondered if older people were just putting a positive spin on their experience or if they reported happiness because they were cognitively impaired. Her research indicated that neither of these reasons were the case.[3]

One major factor that does explain why older people are happy according to Carstensen, is that they realize they are not going to live forever. This actually has a positive impact. They realize the time is now to do what they may have put off. They invest in emotionally meaningful activities and say "no" more often to things they don't enjoy. They begin to live in the moment. She says you could say that old people live like there's no tomorrow.

In another study of people of all ages, Carstensen's findings showed that the emotional aspects of life improve with age, too. Participants were paged five times a day at random moments for several weeks and were asked how happy, sad, and frustrated they felt at that moment. Older people reported as many positive emotions as younger people but far fewer negative ones. Stress, worry, and anger all decrease with age. Carstensen calls these findings about happiness the paradox of aging. It seems that older people gain some capability to deal with loss and unpleasant realities. They are more comfortable than younger people mourning when people they love die and being able to experience sadness. They are more able to see the injustice in the world and be compassionate rather than despairing.[4]

Carstensen also learned that older people remember positive images better than negative images. It seems their brains evolve as they age. Their amygdala, the part of the brain that triggers emotions, was more reactive when they looked at positive images, such as pictures of happy people compared to frowning or angry ones, than when they looked at negative ones. So their positive attitude is actually, at least in part, the result of information from their brain.[5]

Norman Vincent Peale, author and proponent of positive thinking, once said, "Happiness consists not of having but of being, not of possessing but enjoying. It is a warm glow of the heart at peace with itself." This is the good news about aging that many younger people do not know about and do not expect; eightysomethings, even with all their problems and health issues, are happier than other age groups; for some it is even the happiest time of their lives.

CONVERSATION STARTERS
- How would you rate your level of happiness nowadays on a scale of one to ten with one being not at all happy and ten being extremely happy? Why did you rate it as you did?
- What small, everyday things bring you joy and how can you do more of them?
- What are your responsibilities now and how do you feel about them?
- Do you feel less anger, stress, and worry than when you were younger? Why do you think that is true?

TIPS FOR FAMILIES
- Remember the paradox of aging and do not assume your eightysomething family member is miserable.
- Provide your eightysomething family member with options and choices according to their abilities to function.
- Find out about if your eightysomething would like some new plants and go with them to get some.
- If your eightysomething family member *is* unhappy, know this is not an inevitable part of aging. They may be depressed and need medication or talk therapy or be living in the wrong setting for them.

CHAPTER 18

AGING WISELY

earing the story of Solomon was the first time I remember someone being described as wise. You probably know the story. Two women come to Solomon, each claiming that the same baby was theirs. They ask him to judge who is the real mother. He calls for a sword, suggesting he will cut the baby in two. One of the women protests, saying, "Give the baby to the other woman." Solomon proclaims that this one must be the real mother. He explains that a mother will do anything to save the life of her child, including giving it to someone else. I learned, then, that being wise was more complicated than compromising, finding the middle ground. It is about good judgment, feelings, and psychological understanding.

Years later as I was interviewing many eightysomethings about what lessons they had learned over their long lives, I realized I still was wondering about wisdom and what it meant to age wisely. I turned to Erik Erikson and Joan Erikson, who laid the groundwork for studies of human development, and to their book, *The Life Cycle Completed*. They see wisdom as a strength that flowers in old age. For each stage of life, they identified a psychological challenge that needs to be successfully met in order to move on to the next stage. The challenge in their eighth stage, old age, is a struggle between integrity and despair. If people can maintain their integrity, then wisdom, the final strength of old age, can flourish. But what exactly is integrity?[1]

Joan Erikson understands integrity as the capacity to hold together, a sense of coherence and wholeness. Despair, on the other hand, is the loss of hope. People are despairing when the inevitable losses at this last stage of life—loss of autonomy, intimacy, and loved ones—overwhelm them and can't be managed. It wins out over integrity when there is a lack of vital involvement, a sense of stagnation, and an awareness there is no time left for change.[2]

I asked the eightysomethings whom I interviewed what lessons they had learned from their long lives about what really matters. Here are some representative comments gleaned from their many responses:

> Live openly, caringly, honestly. Don't close up. Be open to every situation. Listen. Don't be judgmental. Get educated. Live in the now. Family is what matters. Most satisfaction comes from serving others. Do good for the world. Work is very important. Spend time and energy for good causes and for the family. Do what you like. Be in contact with a higher power. Do what you dream. Notice what is happening in the present. Help others. Love one another. Be true to oneself. Live the right way—don't drink, don't smoke. Be busy. Don't worry about money. Enjoy each day. Live sustainably. Live in the now. Let go. Anger doesn't accomplish anything. Follow your own path. No drugs and no tattoos or drinking to excess. Be honest. Good relationships are what matter. Be concerned about others. Help others live better. Family. Religion is important. No need to achieve. Be kind. Walk a mile a day. Preserve the Universe.

I identified five themes in this jumble: the importance of family, following your dreams, serving others, living in the present, and remembering that relationships matter. A few people focused on God and religion and a few on moralistic prescriptions. But what no one mentioned is success, accomplishments, power, fame, and looking good. Isn't it interesting that, although our culture is obsessed with getting ahead and material things, that no one thinks those are, finally, what really matters?

There was another set of comments from those people who were unhappy, comments that sounded like they had given up hope:

> It's time to go. I am slowly declining. I ruminate about disasters all the time. How long am I going to last? I am not happy. I don't know if I am better off dead or alive. I avoid people; most of them don't know enough and they are boring. The state of the world distresses me, I am glad that I will not be around to see it all happen. My life is miserable, I am stuck here.

But these despairing comments came from a very few people. Of those I interviewed, only eleven of the 128, or about 9 percent, described themselves as unhappy. The overwhelming majority of those I interviewed were happy. It must be acknowledged, they were on the whole, more educated and better off financially, than the average eighty-year-old person in the United States. Almost a half of those living in nursing homes were unhappy. They of course were living with major health issues.

I do want to emphasize, however, that despair in old age is not inevitable. Some unhappy people are actually clinically depressed and need medication. Others are lonely and need more social support and wise counsel to help them adapt to their circumstances. Some despairing people need a higher level of care or a move to a different environment because of their health.

As I thought about the wisdom of eightysomethings, it was clear to me that most of us will not go down in the history books like George Washington or Lady Gaga. But still many of us may want to have a way to pass on to our children, grandchildren, and future generations what we have learned in our long lives about what is most important and what we stood for. We may also want to share with our grandchildren our thoughts and dreams for them as they pass certain important life thresholds such as graduating from high school or getting married. And it is very possible we may not be there to celebrate with them. Writing a legacy letter is a wonderful way for eightysomethings to do these things. It doesn't have to be a long memoir or a complicated process. The letter can be as short as a single page and yet can be truly meaningful. See Appendix II for a template for help with writing such a letter. I have also included several actual letters to a specific family member on the occasion of a graduation, a marriage, and a birth. These examples can help you get started in writing your own legacy letters and you are welcome to use any parts of them that you like in your own letters.

I realized it is not only the lessons that elders have learned that are important for younger generations, but also, just as important, are the models they can provide to us for how to live wisely in the last stage of life. I have chosen four people who, living in very different kinds of situations, impressed me as an eightysomething who is aging wisely.

First, there is Pauline, eighty-six, who lives in a nursing home in Massachusetts. She *holds together*, to use the Eriksons' term, despite the direst of circumstances. A staff person at the nursing home where she lives told me, "Be sure and interview Pauline, she is special." I was somewhat taken aback, therefore, when I met Pauline to find out that she was totally blind, severely hearing-impaired, and in a wheelchair. Pauline looked like a bird with a plume of white hair. Her sightless eyes were clouded, a milky blue, and her tiny body, childlike, and her arms like sticks. *Special?* I asked myself. *Really?*

I moved closer to Pauline to speak, raising my voice so she could hear, almost shouting. She told me she was the mother of six children, five boys and a girl. She is so happy they live around here and all come to see her frequently except one son who is a truck driver. His schedule is busy, she explained—forgiving his neglect but not glossing over his absence. She wishes he would come.

When she didn't hear my next question, she asked me to repeat it, two more times, until she did. She didn't pretend to hear as so many deaf people do. I was impressed by her authenticity. Pauline told me she has been blind for three years and misses reading terribly. Even though she doesn't hear at all well, she loves music, and every now and then she catches some on the TV or radio. What makes her really happy is the recent birth of a first great-grandchild. His name is Bobby. She can't wait for his parents to bring him for a visit.

Pauline's ability to care about this baby, whom she will never see grow up, and to focus on someone other than herself, is impressive. Not everyone with her circumstances would be able to do that. Pauline remains whole, no matter how limited her life. Special, yes.

Miriam, eighty-one, whose life has been far more comfortable than Pauline's, did not strike me at first as particularly wise. But as I learned about her ability to manage the everyday activities of life and adapt to change, I saw her mettle.

She began, "When I was in my teens we lived in Memphis and it was all so clear to me how my life would unfold. I would go to college, get married to someone who was Jewish, and have children. I grew up in a kosher home with lots of aunts and uncles living nearby. I, like my parents, was committed to a Jewish way of life. Part of this was strict morals—I wouldn't sleep with a guy, kiss on the first date, and I would never get drunk." She never even thought of having a career.

Her predictions of her life played out as planned until she moved from Tennessee to southeastern Texas shortly after her marriage. Suddenly she had to make a world for herself away from family. She joined a conservative synagogue to find a like-minded community. Two children came quickly, one after the other.

When the kids were in school, Miriam went to work in a small business and a few years later went back to school part time and got a business degree. She changed as she encountered new ideas. She saw firsthand how others, outside her Jewish community, lived. Her world opened up. She began to read the newspaper and to become active in local politics.

Now, retired, Miriam stays busy. She participates in several book groups and plays bridge and mahjong. "My husband and I go out to lunch every day and have our little routines. We like movies and lectures and in our sixties and seventies we traveled a lot. If I stay home all day it bothers me," she said.

Two events shattered Miriam's life this year. First, her home was flooded during a hurricane. She never imagined she would ever move from her home of twenty-six years, but that changed when four inches of water suddenly sloshed into the house. A neighbor learned about their plight from a post on Facebook. A few minutes later he came by in a kayak to rescue them and they never got back. They sold their house *as is* and a few months later moved to a condo.

"The other shattering event happened just yesterday," she told me during out interview. "My husband who has COPD went on oxygen. They brought in these big machines. Now he doesn't know if he can go on our trip to see my sister or whether he can ever go to the movies again. I keep telling him, 'We will figure it out'." Miriam continued, "These last few weeks, I began having some funny thoughts. About things I might want to do in the future. Things I want to try. I am mechanical and I want to do something with that talent."

"What have I learned in my life that I want to pass on to my grandchildren? I want them to give back. They have so much money compared to how I grew up and I just hope they aren't spoiled. I hope they have some caring for the world and I hope they stay connected to Judaism. And I want them to look out for each other. My mother taught me and my sister that we should stay close. And we have," Miriam said.

I am impressed by how well Miriam has lived her life. Although she has been through a sudden and traumatic loss of her house, she is adjusted to the new condo. She has adapted gracefully to growing old and now becoming a caretaker. At the same time, she has never abandoned her values or wavered from her commitment to a Jewish way of life. She has skillfully managed her everyday life from the smallest details to the bigger picture items. Although there are things like the flood and her husband's illness that she can't control, she remains confident that she can figure it out.

Miriam is beginning to take stock of her life and to have some "funny little thoughts." I wonder if she may see that being so busy has meant that she has been missing some of the pleasures of old age.

Zed, eighty-four, is a lifelong New Yorker whose greatest pleasure now is giving lectures. He was never much of a student and went right to work in a garment factory after high school. He married and had a child. In his late forties, while still a manager in a factory, he got a master's degree in American history at night and found that, "history was my thing." From that point, his life expanded in many directions all at once. He taught courses on the American Civil War and the presidents at a nearby YMCA. He retired from the factory and began teaching in Florida in the winters. Not only history but also courses on baseball and genealogy. He has been happiest when lecturing and seeing that his audience is enthralled. He had loved Sir Arthur Conan Doyle's Sherlock Holmes books for years and now is active in a Sherlock Club. He translated letters from his grandfather in Lithuania and sent them to the family.

His wife died twenty years ago and he was alone for many years. Three years ago, he met a woman through a dating site, Single Booklovers, that goes back before the Internet. They started by writing letters to each other. When they actually met, Zed said he had never laughed so much in his life. They fell madly in love and now they have moved in together. They will spend the rest of their lives together.

Zed told me what he has learned over his many years is that you need to find out what you love to do: "Don't complain, do what you enjoy." It seems that in the second half of his life he found what it was that he loved.

Part of wisdom is self-knowledge. He also had the courage to act on that knowledge. And that courage is another part of wisdom.

Diantha, eighty-eight and living in New Jersey, started out life with a plan similar to Miriam's—marriage and children. As a child she felt like a misfit, that she had been born into the wrong family. She remembers deciding she would never let her critical mother know who she really was. Diantha did marry young and have children, but her pathway, like Miriam's and Zed's, took an unexpected turn. When she was in her forties she went into training to become a Jungian analyst. Training included years of analysis, supervision, as well as academic courses.

In one analysis session she shared her dream about a four-year-old girl locked in a closet. The little girl, sitting inside, had the key. Diantha left her therapy session and went to sit on a bench in Central Park. As she pondered what her dream might have to tell her, she experienced a wave of peacefulness flow through her body. She felt very alive. "Everything suddenly came together inside me, the connection of psyche, soul, and body. I was whole," she said. "And for the rest of my life I have wanted to give my patients that same experience of wholeness that I had sitting on that bench. I wanted to help them lead their lives from the heart rather than from the head. I wanted them to be at ease with their bodies."

Diantha worked with that image of the little girl for many months. Her analyst asked her to draw a series of pictures of the little girl growing older year by year. As the pictures changed, Diantha was learning to mother the inner little girl who was herself. "I was doing what had been left undone by my real mother. My mother did everything but mother. The hardest lesson I had to learn was that in some ways I was actually like my mother."

When she became an analyst, Diantha focused on touch and body-work as part of the way she worked with people. Most therapists back then didn't touch anyone she explained. She learned how to do bodywork from Ilana Rubenfeld, who pioneered the integration of emotions, intuition, and bodywork into psychotherapy. In our world that usually separates mind and body, she saw they were the same, interconnected.

Diantha has slowed down in her late eighties. She is still working with a few patients but is also caring for her husband who has a medical condition. She tells me they were having sex until three years ago, but that it is no longer possible. That has been a huge loss for them. "What is special for me now is time with my grandchildren—just being with them in ways I could never be with my own children because I was so busy doing."

Diantha's experience of wholeness and integrity sitting on the park bench was a dramatic epiphany. She has held onto that sense of wholeness and is facing aging and death with equanimity. She is wise. To get to that wisdom took a certain boldness and ongoing reflection on her experiences. She learned how to get help to move past her wounds of childhood and to chart a new course for her life.

Of course we don't all need years of therapy or a fancy education to learn and to be wise. Wise people can be found in every corner of the world and at every level of education. It frequently is said that experience is the best teacher. But I have learned that is not the whole truth. You do not learn from your experience unless you reflect on it. I end this chapter with a quote from Virginia Woolf: "The compensation of growing old, Peter Walsh thought, coming out of Regent's Park, and holding his hat in hand, was simply this; that the passions remain as strong as ever, but one has gained—at last!—the power which adds the supreme flavour to existence—the power of taking hold of experience, of turning it round, slowly, in the light."[3]

CONVERSATION STARTERS
- What was your life plan at twenty and in what ways did your life stick to the plan and in what ways did it go in different directions?

- Do you find yourself doing more reflecting on what you have learned in your life than at earlier times? Have you considered writing a Legacy Letter? (See Appendix II for more about these).
- What has helped you cope in moments of despair?
- What keeps you engaged in the present and what are you looking forward to in the future?

TIPS FOR FAMILIES

- Ask your eightysomething what are the most important lessons they have learned over their long life.
- If your eightysomething seems down in the dumps and depressed most of the time, see if you can get them evaluated for depression by a doctor or psychiatrist. They may need medications to feel better.
- Work with your eightysomething to develop a way for them to share their wisdom, stories, and experience with the younger generation. Many families have found that it works well to interview them about their life and record the interview. For example, one college-age grandchild interviewed her grandfather three Monday nights in a row for an hour and then wrote up the interviews for the family. Joining a writing groups or a memoir groups are great ways to get this done.
- Suggest they write a Legacy Letter where on a page or two they write down their thoughts about what really matters for their kids and future generations. See Appendix II for a template on how to do this. See if you can help them with this project.

CHAPTER 19

THE LUCKY GENERATION

I t rained on my Commencement Day at Smith College, June 3, 1956, forcing us inside. Our speaker was a Harvard professor and Pulitzer Prize–winning writer and poet, Archibald MacLeish. A little ho-hum I thought. Not as exciting as last year's speaker, Adlai Stevenson who had made a run for the presidency in 1952. My classmates and I were decked out in our rumpled black robes that we had been wearing around campus for months, as was Smith's tradition.

MacLeish began his speech by characterizing young people in the last few decades in the United States. The twenties were "one long jazz-lit midnight. . . . Half of every college class were stockbrokers and the other half didn't bother." The thirties were "when next to nobody was rich and a great many had nothing at all to do and almost as many had less than they should have had to eat." And he remarked that World War II took "most of the decade of the forties with it."

Then he asked, "What are the fifties like? What are they really like?" He began a shocking description of our generation. He wondered, "Whether the fifties are anything more than a kind of time out, a between-times, a limbo, an interim epoch to be occupied by an interim generation, a Gaza strip of unhistory to be lived." More alarmingly, he said, "The fifties are years without describable faces." He concluded that they were "a period in which things are not to be done, but a period in which things are to be kept from being done."[1]

I was stunned, upset, and shamed. What was this man saying? Was I, and my cohort of young people, really an interim generation with blank faces, not doing things? It was a jolt of awareness that I have never forgotten. It made me feel that my generation was being judged and invalidated. MacLeish was not alone when he described my generation negatively. The phrase, the Silent Generation, had first appeared in an article in *Time* magazine in 1951 that had labeled us "unimaginative" and "cautious."[2] The Silent Generation label has stuck and to this day makes me sad and annoyed. I bristle when discussions of our generation are short or nonexistent, sandwiched between glowing praise for the Greatest Generation and lengthy comments about the Baby Boomers.

Elwood Carlson's 2008 book, *The Lucky Few,* presents a different and a far more positive picture of our generation than MacLeish did back in 1956. Carlson, a sociology professor at Florida State University with expertise in quantitative research, sees those born between 1929 and 1944 as being an extraordinarily fortunate generational cohort that he calls the "Lucky Few." Now in their seventies and eighties, they, like me, have lived their adult lives mostly in peacetime with prosperity and unparalleled stability. Over sixty years, I began to see all the upsides of living during these years and, gradually, have revised my view of my generation from being cautious and unimaginative to having been born under a lucky star.

The Baby Boomers, unlike the Lucky Few, have been in the limelight their entire lives. The birth rate in the United States exploded in 1946 after the end of the World War II. It reached a high of 4.3 million births a year compared to high of 2.5 million in the generation before them. The Baby Boomers have been labeled selfish, narcissistic, materialistic and socially responsible—quite different from the usual descriptions of the Silent Generation. They experienced the sexual revolution, the Civil Rights Movement, the Womens' movement—major societal upheavals. The Boomers are now at retirement age and they start turning eighty in 2026.[3] Although they will bring their unique experiences as they deal with old age, they have much to learn from previous generations of eigh-tysomethings. Although the historical background changes over time, the psychological tasks of aging remain essentially unchanged.

The Silent Generation has lived in propitious times and flourished beyond our wildest dreams. Carlson's *The Lucky Few* provided me with the statistics and facts to back up this point of view.

The Lucky Few generation was smaller than the one before and the one that followed it. During the Great Depression and war years when they were born, many of the couples who were their parents postponed having a family or planned a small family. There were about a third fewer babies born in the Lucky Few generation than in the previous one.[4] Growing up with parents who had skimped and saved for many years, most of this generation grew up with a scarcity mentality and worked hard as chil-dren. Twenty-five percent of them grew up on farms compared to 9 per-cent of Baby Boomers. For the Lucky Generation who wanted to go to college, there seemed to be no problem at all in gaining admission if one had the funds. And when it was time to go to work, most found jobs easily.

Most of the Lucky Generation grew up in intact families with a mother and a father and several siblings, more siblings that the usual family today. The Lucky Few themselves when they became parents had more babies than their parents. On average there were 3.3 births compared to 3.0 for their parents' generation and 2.8 for the Boomers. Divorce was still out of the ordinary. Most mothers did not work outside the home. And while there were many shot gun weddings in the fifties, it was not widely accepted. Many pregnant girls were sent away for months to visit relatives and their babies were given up for adoption.

Over half of the males in the Lucky Generation served in the armed services and all of them lived with the draft. The large majority of those in the armed services, however, served in peacetime and stayed in the United States. There were casualties in Korea, but nothing like the losses in World War II. Most veterans found jobs easily when they left the service.

The Lucky Generation married young. At one point the average bride was younger than twenty. They have been the most-married generation, with 95 percent of women marrying at some point in their lives. And in the post-war prosperity, they had many children. By age twenty-five, two-thirds of women in the Lucky Few Generation had become mothers compared to about half of them for the generation before and after.

According to Carlson, the Lucky Few have less respect for key social institutions and authority than previous generations but more than recent generations.[5] More of them started out as Republicans than in the generations before and after. More of them believe that "most people try to be fair" than all succeeding generations.

In some ways, African Americans in the Lucky Few generation shared in the luck, making more progress in education and prosperity than previous generations, but they did not move ahead at the same rate as their white counterparts as segregation persisted in many realms with devastating results.[6]

The stories of Francis, Lizzie, and Joel, three of the 128 eightysomethings whom I interviewed, showcase many of the characteristics that are typical of the Lucky Few generation. They also highlight the uniqueness of the times in which they lived. The experiences of ordinary people like them make clear how the trends and statistics that differentiate this generation from all the others have played out.

Francis, eighty, a tanned, handsome, moon-faced man who radiates well-being, grew up in North Carolina and now lives in New Orleans. His much older brother, who was a pilot in the 8th Air Force during World War II, was his lifelong hero. He filled Francis's mind with exciting stories of his fourteen missions over Germany and other experiences during the war.

After college, Francis enlisted in the Navy where he was commissioned as a lieutenant. During the Cuban Missile Crisis, he was on a ship out of Key West. He admitted, "It was pretty scary. We followed a Russian ship and we ran patrols off shore. But no one ever fired at me. I dodged the war bullet just by the virtue of my age, being too young for the war."

Later Francis was transferred to New Orleans where he has lived ever since. He left the military because it didn't pay enough and within days found a job at IBM and a local girl he would marry. After decades with IBM, when he was fifty-six, he was offered a buyout; it was just too good a deal to refuse, so he retired. After that, he consulted part-time and then went to work briefly as a dealer at a famous New Orleans Casino. It was fun until they promoted him to be in charge of a whole table and he quit because it was too much responsibility. Now he plays golf two or three times a week, reads a lot of history books, and volunteers one day a week at the Museum of World War II. He is still happily married and is thrilled that his two kids live nearby.

Francis feels he has coasted through his whole life, experiencing few struggles. Living in the shadow of his brother and World War II, he is a bit embarrassed that he enjoyed the safety of being in the military in peacetime and how easy it was to find a good job that provided him and his family with a comfortable life. At eighty, he has already been retired for twenty-four years, living well on his still-secure pension. He has certainly been lucky.

Lizzie's life story, like that of Francis, reflects amazing continuity. Lizzie grew up in southern Connecticut. She recalls her childhood as idyllic and carefree. She and her brothers and sisters rode their bikes around town going hither and yon without a second thought of safety, just being sure to show up for dinner. Three of her siblings are alive today, two brothers age eighty-nine and ninety-two and a sister who is a seventy-seven. They have always played a huge role in her life. She was a bridesmaid at each of their weddings. As adults, all of the brothers and sisters would gather at their parents' house for Christmas, Easter, Memorial Day, and Labor Day.

She started by telling me she was still grieving the death of her sister Mary, who died four years ago: "Her death really knocked me for a loop." They always lived close to each other and visited back and forth with their grandkids for weekends when they didn't live in the same town. She believes the brothers and sisters were so close because of her dad. He assigned chores and held each child to them. Every day after breakfast they gathered in the living room for morning prayers. Then their father would improvise some prayers, but he always remembered the needy in their town and the two missionaries he supported, one in India and one in Greece.

Lizzie now lives with her husband Jack in a retirement community in Hartford, Connecticut. At eighty-seven, Lizzie is a pretty woman with limpid blue eyes, a girlish manner, and a breathless quality to her speech. Lizzie and Jack lived in a suburb of Hartford for more that forty years. Jack has worked his entire life for the same insurance company. Once her kids were launched, Lizzie taught math for twenty-five years at the same middle school. They have remained members of the same church for fifty years.

Today both Lizzie and Jack have multiple health issues and make many trips each year to the hospital. But she is not a complainer. She feels grateful to be able to afford such a nice retirement community and so grateful that she and Jack have each other. She said, "Even though I don't see my brothers and sister all that often now, they are there."

When I reflect on Lizzie's life, the stability she has experienced is remarkable. Same town for forty years, same church for fifty years, Jack working at the same company his entire life. A posse of brothers and sisters that has stayed connected since childhood and grown old together. I think of the contrast with my young clients who are all so worried about their futures: getting a job, paying their college loans, and deciding whether or not to have a family. They cannot begin to imagine the kind of security Lizzie has felt throughout her life or the lack of ambivalence she has felt about her role and work/life balance. Almost all young women today seem to be riddled with guilt and feeling of uncertainty whether they are single or married, work outside the home or are a stay-at-home wife.[7] But yet, I think those in this current generation might wonder if Lizzie hasn't missed out on something important having such stability and continuity in her life.

Joel's early life, compared to Francis and Lizzie's, was anything but stable or lucky. His life didn't turn around until he was in his fifties. His story illustrates the serious problems that some of the Lucky Generation faced in their families that were never talked about and never addressed. In Joel's case, his father was an alcoholic and his mother mentally ill. His only brother was a deeply troubled child. Joel himself was an anxious kid, always worried that there would be trouble at home or that he would fail at school. He was bullied for several months by other second graders.

Joel grew up in a suburb of Philadelphia. His parents were Republican and Jewish. "Republican first and Jewish second," he explained. "I was brought up to be secular and assimilated. I had something sort of resembling a Bar Mitzvah, a party, but I never learned any Hebrew."

In ninth grade, Joel was sent away to a conservative all-boys boarding school in New Jersey where, as a Jew, he said, he didn't quite fit in: "A few of my classmates were blatantly anti-Semitic." Once he came back to his room to find it messed up, with his mattress and his books thrown out the window. Two signs had been taped to the door. *You are a dirty Jew* and *I hate Jews*. The school made a pro forma attempt to figure out who had done it, but their efforts fizzled quickly. Someone told Joel which boy was guilty and Joel confronted him. But Joel "just felt worse because I didn't punch him out."

In Joel's twenties it didn't get any better. While he was in the service for three years, his parents divorced, his brother committed suicide, and Joel rushed into an early marriage that was a disaster from the start.

At this point Joel decided he had to do something constructive with his life and a few months later applied to medical school. With his up and down grades, he was surprised that one school accepted him. About that time he got divorced and then quickly remarried. Regrettably, his second marriage was also unhappy. Then his wife fell ill with cancer and she died after a two-year struggle. Joel was left with four small children to raise.

From then on, things in Joel's life began to get better. His kids did fine. He became a successful doctor. He married a woman whom he adored. Joel has now been married thirty years to his third wife. "I am happy beyond anything I could ever have imagined," he told me. Today he is quite healthy and extremely busy. At eighty-three, he still practices medicine and does some teaching. He has run seven marathons and still runs most days. He has written a book of short stories and sings in a chorale. He wound up our interview by saying, "Finally, I learned how to love and how to be happy. It is still hard for me to believe."

Joel's life ran counter to many of the trends and norms that characterize the Lucky Few generation. No intact family, and no security. With a mentally ill mother and brother, divorced parents, and high level of anxiety himself, it was a tough beginning. It is a small miracle that he could experience such a remarkable change of fortune and to be thriving so magnificently at eighty-three. He told me he was helped along the way by a lot of therapy. I believe, also, that his years of therapy helped him heal from the trauma of his childhood. This was lucky because many men are not able to ask for the help they need. I believe he was also aided by the fact he was living in a peaceful and prosperous world that provided lots of opportunities for change and second chances.

Most eightysomethings today do not feel like they have been an interim generation or a faceless generation. Their lives have been filled with events, changes, and actions. But there is a sense that many of us were swept along in the wave of the post-war culture. We did seek normalcy—family, job, security—more than adventure, change, or career success. And the

Baby Boomers have had their own journey and may feel misunderstood as well. But all generations basically face the same fundamental psychological tasks as eightysomethings: managing loss and letting go.

My story. I was of my time, too. My goals were simply marriage and a big, happy family. By the time I graduated from college and heard Archibald MacLeish's address, I was already married. No thoughts of a career or even a job. So it was a shock when I had trouble getting pregnant. In spite of some infertility problems and three miscarriages, by thirty-two I had my big family—four boys, one of whom we adopted.

But my dreams changed after I went to work—a part-time teaching job. I was totally surprised to discover how much I loved working. Now fulfillment meant my kids *and* a job.

And I kept on evolving. Before long I had enrolled in a program to get a social work degree. I realized how much I also liked going to school as well. When I finished my social work program, I went to work as a psychotherapist in a community mental health center. After ten years there I went back to graduate school again, this time to get a PhD in social psychology. In my next phase, I worked in a management consulting firm, after a few years starting my own firm with two other women. I loved this work, too. It took me to corporations and organizations around the globe. For example, I went to Bangladesh ten times to facilitate large group strategic planning sessions for UNICEF. Clearly, my life was no longer on the beaten path. I felt very lucky and I knew, also, that I had worked hard to find my niche in the world.

Many of us in my generation did live conventional lives. And, really, how lucky that is, too. But many others have explored all kinds of alternative lifestyles and vocations. Most of us have shared in the good luck. We have had the chance to live out our lives in a time of mostly peace, mostly prosperity, mostly safety, and much opportunity. This was different for the previous generation and, sadly, also different for many in the generations that have followed.

CONVERSATION STARTERS

- In what ways do you see your generation as being lucky? Unlucky?
- In what ways do you see your own life as being lucky?
- What do you want your grandchildren and the younger generation to know about the world you grew up in?
- What do you want them to know about what you think matters most?

TIPS FOR FAMILIES

- Schedule some time to interview your eightysomething about the most interesting events they have experienced that they would like the future generations to know about.
- Help your eightysomething write a Legacy Letter. It is much more likely to get done if you get involved. See Appendix II. for a template.
- Growing up before the social revolutions of the late sixties shaped the views of most of today's eightysomethings. Find out how their attitudes about Civil Rights, sex, and the women's movement have changed over the years.

CHAPTER 20

A NEW VISION OF OLD AGE

L ife expectancy in Hong Kong is an amazing 84.3 years, the longest of any city in the world. This compares to a life expectancy of seventy-nine years in the United States. And despite horrific pollution in Hong Kong which affects many people each year. It is ironic, because the name Hong Kong means "Fragrant Harbor." A short video, "Why This Polluted Asian City Has the Greatest Life Expectancy" explains the reasons.[1]

Key factors explaining the longevity include the frequency of daily contacts because of the density of Hong Kong, the moderate climate, the typical diet that has ample amounts of fresh fish, fruits, and vegetables, and the well-developed and affordable public transportation system. The city also has miles of walkways, and mountains and beaches are both close by and accessible. There is healthcare for all, and fewer people in the city smoke than in many places, only 10 percent. You have to wonder, if Hong Kong solved its pollution problems, how much further would average life expectancy be extended?

More people in the United States are also living longer than ever before in any time in our history, though less long than in Hong Kong. In the time of Thomas Jefferson, only half the population lived to be eighteen. In 1930, life expectancy was less than sixty, while today it is 81.2 years for women and 76.4 years for men. Women who reach eighty can expect to live on average for an additional 9.1 years, and men for seven years. And the good news is that many of them will live in relatively good health.

But what is the purpose of living all those years after sixty-five when most people are no longer working? What do the very old contribute to society? What are the real possibilities for people at this stage of life? These are the important questions that I tackle in this chapter.

Becca Levy, professor of epidemiology and psychology at Yale University, has found in her research that aging is often viewed as a physical process of deterioration and decline. Old people are seen as useless, slow, and confused more often than they are seen as confident, wise, and accomplished. Attitudes toward old people are formed in childhood and internalized at an early age. And it is ironic that if a person is lucky to live long enough, they eventually become one of those old people. And then they have to deal with their own bias, their ageism, toward people like themselves.

As people age, any negative views and assumptions about old people they have may be reinforced by cues from their experience. This happens when older people are denied employment, when they are no longer chosen for roles with influence and power, when they are ignored, and when they are patronized. Many eightysomethings come to believe that their role is to get out of the way of the action, to be invisible and not to be a burden on their children. They come to think they should be positive and uncomplaining as they sit on the sidelines.

Prejudice against the old is different from other forms of bias because it is one area that has not yet been declared out of bounds by some of the political correctness enforcers. People can say things like, "We need younger leaders," and "The older people should make room for the younger generation." And no one calls them out.

Of course, the negative attitudes toward the elderly are not the whole story. This chapter is also about a more positive vision of old age, one that is hopeful and feasible. Part of the hope comes from new research about the brain and its ability to heal, grow, and develop over time. This process is called neuroplasticity. It means that our fate is not sealed. Much of how our aging unfolds depends on ourselves, our attitudes, and our behavior.

Yet the impact today of negative attitudes about aging can be immense. Becca Levy's research indicates that people who harbored negative attitudes of aging in their younger life can double their risk of having a cardiovascular event and other health issues as they age. On the other hand, people with positive self-perceptions of aging live 7.5 years longer than others.[2] These findings ought to be a wake-up call about the need to revise our attitudes about aging.

Levy also makes clear that aging is far more than the physiological process of decline. More importantly, it is a social construct. That means that how people age can be changed over time if they receive education and training and if both their attitudes and their behaviors are modified. Many of our institutions, our laws, and our policies are built on assumptions about the old, assumptions that are outdated and, in some cases, false. They need to be modified to reflect newer understandings of the aging process.

As most people age into their eighties today, they are in no way prepared to resist the widely accepted, albeit outdated, views of what older people are supposed to do. I can speak from my own experience about that because when I was approaching sixty-five, I came smack up against the conventional thinking about retirement.

I was the managing partner at Ibis Consulting Group, a firm that focused on promoting diversity and increasing effectiveness in organizations. Working there was going well for me and was highly satisfying. However, for several years many friends and acquaintances had been asking me repeatedly, "What are you going to do after you retire?" My husband had retired at sixty-two. I began thinking, it must be time for me to leave. Sixty-five is when you retire, isn't it? That's just the way it was then.

But then one day it dawned on me, I don't want to retire. I had been a full-time mom for nine years, so I always felt I had a late start in my career. I had left the usual patterns for women in my time and in my social group when I went to work full time as a mother of four, when I wrote a book about Gypsies, when I got a PhD at age fifty. Gradually, I realized that I didn't have to stop this work that I love. I needed to trust my own experience. I remembered that the idea of retirement at sixty-five came from the fact that this was the age when you could start collecting social security. But that was in the 1930s, when half the people were dead by sixty-five.

So I just kept on working at my job. And flourishing. I finally left Ibis when I was seventy-five. By then the marketing and the travel were becoming a burden to me and it felt like the right time to go. It was a painless transition, partly because I planned to go back right away to my psychotherapy practice. I had always renewed my social work license and the option to return to clinical work. Psychotherapy was a wonderful fit for me in my seventies, and continues to be for me in my eighties, despite my diminished energy. At eighty-four, I see fewer clients.

We all age at our own pace. Not all eightysomethings, in fact, only a few of us, actually want to work. And many people now and in the future will have to work longer than they would like. But it is so important that those of us who do have the desire to work be able to do it.

And aging is not just about individual behavior and beliefs; we must think about supporting the needs of all types and kinds of older people as a group. We need new solutions that create a high-quality environment for all ages. Our communities are integrated social systems where the well-being of one segment of the community affects all parts.

And communities are catching on. Some of them are trying to understand the needs of their older residents. Salem, Massachusetts, for example, a small city of forty-three thousand people, formed a leadership team to explore making their city more age-friendly. Their first action step was to conduct a survey of everyone over fifty in the city. Some of their responses were surprising. To the question, "Do you feel the thoughts and opinions of older adults are valued in Salem?" the majority, some 63 percent of respondents, said "no" or "not sure." Other comments like those below opened their eyes to the fact that there were some serious issues for the older people in their city.

> We don't want to be segregated.
> Help me feel useful.
> Stop treating over 60s as non-existent and unnecessary, as if they have no mind or good judgment.
> The city squanders the knowledge of older people.
> It is important not to isolate older folks from younger folks.[3]

Later in this chapter, I share Salem's action plan to address the concerns that they identified. But now I turn to Orca, an eightysomething woman with few resources and without much support from family. Her story suggests what life can be like for old people living alone in the United States and the kinds of issues they face.

Orca was a single mom who raised two sons. She worked in a florist shop for many years. Now she lives alone in a small apartment twenty miles north of Boston. Her annual income comes entirely from her social security check.

Orca told me about her present life:

> I have had two strokes, am on a walker, and I have macular degeneration. I tell my sons, "You have no idea what's coming down the road for you." Neither of them takes care of me. One son drops off a bunch of frozen dinners every two weeks or so and I warm them in the microwave. I do cold cuts for lunch. My friend cuts my hair and a neighbor fixes my pills for me. I can't drive and I don't know a lot of people. So I don't have any fun. When I feel down, I try and call my cousin or my other

friend. It is not like when I was a kid and could run out at night and jump rope or play hopscotch with a bunch of kids. I don't go out, I just watch TV. It's not easy.

What impresses me about Orca is that she has been able to persuade people—friends and family—to provide her with what she needs to survive. Sure, she is cranky and a complainer, but where are the services and support systems from her town? It seems no one is checking in on her. It will be so easy for her to fall between the cracks. And what is also upsetting, no one is keeping her company. She is terribly lonely.

Orca's story of living alone took me first to the research on loneliness. Julianne Holt-Lunstad, a professor of psychology at Brigham Young University, says that we are in the middle of a loneliness epidemic and it is only getting worse.[4] In Great Britain they have appointed a Minister of Loneliness to deal with their own epidemic.

Loneliness is different from being alone or solitary and affects people who are married as well as single as well as those who may have networks of friends and family. It is a subjective experience, a deep sense of disconnection from other people. Loneliness is all about feelings. It includes feelings of emptiness, and can sometimes include feelings of worthlessness, lack of control, and anger. Loneliness is not the same as depression. You can be lonely and not depressed, and you can be depressed and not lonely.

Holt-Lunstad's research indicated that loneliness is a predictor of premature death. Those who are lonely are twice as likely as others to die from heart disease and Alzheimer's than those who do not feel lonely. They are twice as likely to die from all causes, even when controlling for age, income, and smoking. Lonely people have less restful sleep, higher blood pressure, and weaker immune systems than others.

There is more. People who are lonely feel worse than others when they are sick. It is a painful state according to John Cacioppo of the University of Chicago and author of *Loneliness: Human Nature and the Need for Social Conn*ection. It can be useful when it acts as a signal, a nudge to people, that they need to make connections to other people in order to feel better. Social connections provide an important scaffold for the self.[5]

Orca's story of neglect from her community also led me to learn more about age-friendly communities and the organizations promoting them. The 2015 World Health Organization World Report on Aging & Health says that an age-friendly world will require a transformation of health systems away from disease-based curative models toward providing integrated care for the whole person. It will need to consider the social, emotional, psychological, physical, and spiritual needs of older adults and include providing ways for the aging population to meet their needs for social connection, meaning, purpose, and interdependency.

The World Health Organization (WHO) Global Network for Age-Friendly Cities and Communities was established to foster exchange of experiences and learning between communities as they endeavor to accomplish this transformation. AARP, the American Association of Retired Persons, an organization of forty million people in the United States has created a framework called "8 Domains of Livability" that can be used by communities interested in becoming more age-friendly. It has also created a process for communities to get certified as an age-friendly community.

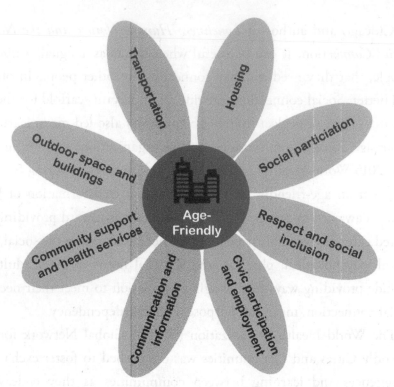

Eight Domains of an Age-Friendly Community
Source: Sandra Harris, Design for Aging Committee, BHA

Some cities like Salem, Massachusetts, that we mentioned earlier in the chapter, have already gone through many steps of this process of certification. Salem's action plan, "Salem for All Ages," was developed by their leadership team. It focuses on aging in place—assisting seniors with maintenance of their homes and encouraging the development of more senior housing options. It also encourages providing more support for family caregivers, expanding access and options for transportation in the city, improving sidewalks and intersections, and supporting the Council on Aging as a focal point for information and support for seniors. The plan also seeks to support social participation and civic engagement of seniors in the city, to encourage age-friendly businesses, and to provide information on volunteer options including work for taxes options. They plan to provide education to all residents about the issues and concerns of aging adults.

Salem is just one of 296 cities and towns in the nation that have participated in the AARP process, a process that takes about five years. New York and Massachusetts have also committed to making their whole state age-friendly. This is an important development as communities strive to offer older people a variety of options and alternatives that did not exist before. For example, there was a recent article in the *Washington Post* reporting that a record number of folks age eighty-five and older are now working—255,000 of them to be more exact.[6]

Theodore Roszak, author of *The Making of an Elder Culture*, believes that the future lies with the old, not only because their numbers are increasing or because their needs have been neglected, but also because of their values. The old can help create a saner, more compassionate, more sustainable world for everyone. The elderly can wean people away from their obsession with youth, with competition, and with the consumption of goods. They can be advocates for the larger public good.

I believe, like Roszak, that elders have a great deal to offer younger generations. They are worthy of attention from the younger generation as keepers of family traditions, storytellers, and carriers of the moral compass. But I also believe that eightysomethings and those even older are deserving unrelated to anything that they might do. They do not need to justify their long lives by continuing to accomplish. They can demonstrate what a person is like who has completed all the stages of life and has had the opportunity to fully develop his or her character. They can show younger generations what aging wisely looks like.

A number of eightysomethings need care. They are not be able to be independent and may not be able to achieve anything at all. And that is the way it should be. It is their turn to be on the receiving end of care. This is payback for their years of being the achievers and the caregivers. All old people, whether they are healthy or need care, can benefit from support systems that allow them to enjoy the wonders of being alive. And this support needs to come from the community and not just the family.

Today, this is just a vision. To promote more positive attitudes about old age, we must educate our people of all ages about the expanding possibilities for the lives of old people and their value. There is a role for schools, for churches, and for government at all levels. To transform our culture, we must support the existing movements and processes to help our cities and communities to become more age-friendly and create new initiatives that do not yet exist.

I close this chapter and end the book with a story from Maggie, who lives alone on a farm and directs plays. You met her in chapter 5, "Holding On and Letting Go." When I interviewed her for a second time in 2018, she told me that she had found a new love, Griffin. They met at a community theater and discovered that they share many interests. They began a series of long conversations and get-togethers.

Last winter she went down to Florida to visit Griffin for two weeks. One day, as Maggie and Griffin parked their car at the beach, there were five young men on motorcycles resting nearby. At eighty-nine, neither Maggie nor Griffin walk well or have good balance, so getting into the water was a complicated process. Griffin hobbled along using two canes and Maggie managed with one cane as they slowly made their way across the sandy beach. When they finally got to the water, Griffin tucked all three canes into his belt and the two of them, arm in arm, walked ever so slowly and ever so gingerly, into the deeper water. For a half an hour they bobbed happily in the ocean, holding each other. Then they slowly began to make their way back to the beach. The five guys were still there. One of them called to them as they passed by, "You know, just watching you two go swimming today has made me look forward to growing old."

Maggie was deeply moved. This unlikely comment from the motorcyclist suddenly illuminated for her the meaning of her present life, a life so full of both love and pain. One of her dreams for her children has always been that they will not be afraid of growing old. And since that day the memory of the motorcyclist's comment comes back to her, keeping her going on days when life seems just so very hard.

What a wonderful vision of old age—that all people might no longer fear growing old and that they might see possibilities for joy and love up to their very last days.

CONVERSATION STARTERS

- How do you believe that eightysomethings contribute to society?
- What kinds of support do you get from your community or state that help you manage and enjoy your life?
- What kind of supports should be in place from the community so all people in their eighties can thrive?
- What is your vision for what life in old age should be like?

TIPS FOR FAMILIES

- Talk with your eightysomething about the positive impact on health and longevity that a positive attitude about aging has. Also explore together the idea that you can choose your attitudes.
- Ask your eightysomething family member about being lonely and what has been helpful to them when they are lonely.
- Do some research on the kinds of opportunities, programs, and services for older people that exist in your community. Check out the library, the Council on Aging, the hospital, and adult education programs for starters.
- Help your eightysomething utilize the programs and services that the community provides.

AUTHOR'S NOTES

RESEARCH METHODOLOGY

I used the snowball sampling technique to recruit subjects for my interviews. I started by listing colleagues, friends, and relatives. I asked each of them for the names of eightysomethings who fit my criteria which were that the people were in their eighties and lucid enough for an interview. Then I asked all those whom I interviewed for more names. And so my list grew over time. My subjects were diverse on many characteristics such as gender, race, religion, ethnicity, level of disability, geography, class, and economic level. I was not looking for a sample that was an exact representation of all people in their eighties in the United States. Rather, I was looking to weight the sample with eightysomethings who were thriving and could illustrate various kinds of lifestyles and possibilities. While a number of those I chose were poor, more of them were middle and upper middle class.

About 50 percent of the interviews I conducted were in person and the others were interview by telephone. I traveled to California, Ohio, Louisiana, Virginia, Connecticut, Rhode Island, New Jersey, Pennsylvania, and New York. Those I interviewed lived in all regions of the United States, although more of them reside in New England than other regions.

ACKNOWLEDGMENTS

First and foremost, I am profoundly appreciative of all those people whom I interviewed for the book, 128 eightysomethings and twenty-six of their adult children. They shared freely about their experiences, their joys, and their sorrows, and opened their hearts to me.

Then many thanks to the experts who deepened my own understanding of aging: Allison Christopher, Sunnita Hanjura, M.D., Sarah Hathaway, Ellen Levinson, Hector Montesino, Mudhumathi Rao, M.D., Marguerite Roach, M.D., Bonnie Wilbur, Patricia Zaido.

I am deeply grateful to all the members of my writing group who generously gave of their time, their ideas, their editing skill, and their feedback: Jeanine Calabria, Sue Curtin, Becky-Sue Epstein, Fran Grigsby, Maile Houlihan, Barbara Lynn-Davis, Marti Thomas, and Elizabeth Townsend.

Thanks also to Peggy Cahill who researched for several chapters and helped with the references. Also thanks to Faxon Green who also helped with research.

I am appreciative of Karen Wollam and Gretchen O'Connor who pulled the manuscript together with great skill and good spirits as we made our way to the end. Much appreciation to Alice Kaufman who spent long hours helping with the Endnotes.

My family was supportive from start to finish. My late beloved husband was there for the early thinking about the book. Thanks to my grandchildren, Jonathan, Thomas, and Sarah, who helped me with some ideas, some research, and some articles. I deeply appreciate the many ways my sons, Dan, Paul, Ben, and Jed, and their wives Elizabeth, Vanda, Raquel, and Andrea, and my cousin Caroline Morse were there for me with love and occasional assistance. Peter Gunness provided day to day support and love this last year.

APPENDIX I

50 EXCITING THINGS FOR EIGHTYSOMETHINGS TO DO*

1. Take dancing lessons
2. Get a new puppy
3. Direct a play
4. Sing in a chorus
5. Learn to play pool
6. Exhibit your photographs
7. Get married
8. Volunteer to canvass for a candidate for political office
9. Learn how to make pottery using a kiln
10. Go skiing
11. Spend a week on a ranch
12. Drive coast to coast in a RV
13. Take boxing lessons
14. Paint for a week with a group of artists
15. Go to Asia on a tour
16. Go sky diving
17. Write a book
18. Find a new love
19. Take a course in your community
20. Teach a course
21. Act in a play
22. See a play on Broadway
23. Volunteer at a local prison
24. Go birding in the mountains of Colombia, South America

25. Help other elderly people with their taxes

26. Take an online course on genealogy

27. Host an event for a political candidate

28. Sell a piece of art that you have created

29. Visit the World War II Museum in New Orleans

30. Collect Civil War memorabilia

31. Volunteer at a soup kitchen

32. Get a job

33. Join the board of a local not for profit organization

34. Go kayaking

35. Make a dining room table

36. Give a lecture

37. Create an indoor garden

38. Play in a quartet

39. Go to Rome

40. Collect folk art in Mexico

41. Make a movie

42. Go sailing

43. Write a memoir

44. Go square dancing

45. Join a drumming group

46. Ride a 21-speed three-wheeled "bicycle"

47. Go to a high school or college reunion

48. Take part in a talent show

49. Take a grandchild for an outing or a trip

50. Host a ninetieth birthday party for a friend

*NOTE: This list is made of of things current eightysomethings are doing. It was compiled from people I interviewed for the book and from eightysomethings I met up with this year.

APPENDIX II

LEGACY LETTERS

A legacy letter is a way to pass on to future generations what you would like them to know about you as well as your hopes and dreams for them. A legacy letter can be written for all your descendants and the future generations of your family. Imagine what a gift it would be for them years from now to know a bit about you and what mattered to you.

Suggested template—A legacy letter can be as simple as just four paragraphs and one or two pages. Here is an outline to use.

1. **Some Facts about Me:**
   My name and birthdate
   Names of my parents, siblings, spouse(s), children, grandchildren

2. **What I Stood For**
   I would like to be remembered for. . . .
   I feel proud that I . . . .

3. **What I Learned during My Life**
   I learned that. . . .
   What matters most in life is to. . . .

4. **Message to Future Generations**
   Some of my dreams for you are. . . .
   Some of my hopes and wishes for the world in the future are. . . .

Possible Additions

Stories that illustrate who you were and what you feel good about that you did in your life.

A section on some objects that are important to you that you will pass on. Explain what they mean to you.

Stories about some of the interesting experiences you had in your life.

Descriptions of special places in your life and why they mattered to you.

SAMPLE LEGACY LETTERS

The three letters below illustrate the concept of a legacy letter written to a specific family member for a specific occasion that you expect will take place in the future. Feel free to use any parts of these letters that you like in letters of your own that you write. Hopefully, they will make it easier for you to get started in what can be such a meaningful gift to a grandchild or other relative.

LETTER FOR THE OCCASION OF A GRANDCHILD'S (CHILD'S, NIECE'S, NEPHEW'S, GODCHILD'S) GRADUATION

Dear Maria,

I am writing this letter in May of 2019 for you to have on the occasion of your graduation from college. I wish I could be there to clap long and loud as you receive your diploma. I would be so proud of you. Since I have some reason to believe I may not be there with you, I am writing this letter now to share a few of my thoughts.

Graduations are wonderful celebrations of accomplishment. To receive a diploma means that you spent hours studying for tests and exams. It means you completed papers and projects. It means you finished untold assignments even when you would have rather been doing something else. That hard work and persistence is worth celebrating.

Education has always been important to our family. My paternal grandfather, your great grandfather, who was a black-smith living on the prairie in North Dakota had seven children. He had the dream of his kids getting the education that he never got. Five of his children, including my father, went on to at least two years of college. My maternal grandmother was also one of seven children, and every single one of them in her family went on from high school to attend college. I myself got a four year scholarship to college and that changed my life forever.

When I graduated from college back in 1957, I had only some vague ideas of what kind of work I would do or what my focus would be. I sensed then that education was terribly important and that has been something I have always found to be true. And as you know, I worked in education my whole career. I hope you, too, will find jobs, a career, and a lifestyle that really work for you.

I remember when you were five years old what a loving and energetic kid you were, and how beautifully you sang even then. You had me in tears at your concert in middle school where you sang a solo. You know I love singing, too, and was in two singing groups well into my eighties. I hope you will sing throughout your life.

And when I was your age, I have to admit I did some foolish things like driving too fast because it never occurred to me that

I could be the one to have a life-changing accident. I can only say how much I want you to stay safe so that you can have the opportunity to grow up, to have a long life, and to grow old.

I hope that you will find a loving partner to share your life journey. And, also, that you encounter some wise people who will help you on your way.

Here are a few things I believe that I want to share with you. Kindness is important. Family is always important. Service to the community and those in need is important. You create your future by the choices you make. What matters most is how well you love in this life.

Your loving grandfather

LETTER FOR THE OCCASION OF A GRANDCHILD'S (CHILD'S, NIECE'S, NEPHEW'S, GODCHILD'S) MARRIAGE

Dear Maya,

I am writing this letter for you to have on the occasion of your marriage since it is quite possible that I may not be able to be with you at the wedding. I am writing this letter now to share a few of my thoughts about marriage from the vantage point of my own long life and fifty-nine years of marriage.

Your decision to marry is probably the most important decision you will make in your entire life. A wedding is truly an event to celebrate when two people love each other and have committed to spending the rest of their lives together.

I was engaged when I was just twenty-one and your grandpa was twenty-seven. We married younger back then. Unbelievably, we had only been on eight dates when we got engaged. Despite how little we knew each other, we both felt certain we were making a good choice. We had the same values and both wanted a big family. We got married three months later in my parent's house on December 21, 1955.

It was a happy marriage for the most part. But it took time and attention and there were some tough times. We had to learn how to speak up and tell each other what was on our minds. And we had to adapt as we changed in some major ways from the people we had been on our wedding day. Having four children changed us both. I evolved over the years being a contented stay-at-home mom to going back to school for a social work degree and then becoming a working mom. That was not so usual back then but I was lucky because your Grandpa was unbelievably supportive.

I want to share a few things I have learned about making a marriage work. It is a lot like a tending a garden. If you do not weed a garden, water it, and prune it, it will not flourish. I learned that you need to take time to focus on just each other and the relationship between the two of you. If you have children this becomes very hard. But taking time, even just a mere three minutes, to really connect, in spite of all the tasks and business of the day, will make a huge difference.

I hope you will have days and years that are gloriously happy. But there will be times when you will encounter setbacks, losses, and disappointments. This is inevitable. Life never follows the plans you have made and our dreams change. When the going gets hard, I hope you will learn, as I did, how to get help for the marriage from a wise mentor or a psychotherapist. Learning how to accept what has happened, to adapt to change, and to be resilient after a loss, these are the skills that will keep you happily married. What matters most is always standing on the side of love.

With love from,
Gran

LETTER FOR THE OCCASION OF A BIRTH OF A BABY (A GRANDCHILD, A GREAT-GRANDCHILD, OR A NIECE'S, NEPHEW'S, OR GODCHILD'S GRANDCHILD)

Dear Asher,

I am writing this letter for you to have on the occasion of the birth of your first child. Since it is quite possible I may not be able to be with you when that time comes, I am writing you now, in 2019, to share a few of my thoughts about being a parent.

I remember holding you the very day that you were born. It was a moment of awe and mystery—a miracle as the births all babies are. You were beautiful, full of promise and possibilities.

The birth of a first child is not only the arrival of a new person in the world, it is also a major transition for you. You now become a parent and with that comes a new role that will last for your lifetime. You lifestyle, your every decision, your pathway will now be influenced by the existence of your tiny, growing, eager-to-live baby. Parenting will take time, effort, patience, and flexibility.

There is a lot of nonsense written on how to be a good parent. My hope is that you don't fall for it that there are a set of rules that if you follow them your child will flourish. Since every baby is different you will have to discover from him or her who your baby is. What is she or he feeling? What do they need? What do they want? Some babies will seem from day one just like people in your family. But others will be unexpected, different, and they will require more patience as a parent. It is a matter of commonsense and learning.

And parenting requires balance. You can't forget you own needs. When I became a parent of four kids, including Uncle Paul who was adopted, it took me awhile to learn that your grandpa and I were still the ones in charge, not the kids. We needed to set the rules of the home and the kids would adapt to them.

Of course, parenting is hard. There will be worries, surprises, sickness, sleepless nights. But also unbelievable joy. Most parents love their kids with a passion that is stronger than all others. I know for me, being a parent has been the highlight of my life. I hope it will be the same for you.

With so much love from,
Gran

ENDNOTES

CHAPTER 1: I AM NOT OLD!

1. United Nations, Department of Economic and Social Affairs, Population Division (2017). *World Population Ageing 2017 - Highlights* (ST/ESA/SER.A/397). Downloaded 3/12/2019 from http://www.un.org/en/development/desa/population/publications/pdf/ageing/WPA2017_Highlights.pdf.

2. "Life Expectancy in North America 2017" downloaded 3/12/2019 from https://www.statista.com/statistics/274513/life-expectancy-in-north-america/.

3. United Nations, Department of Economic and Social Affairs, Population Division (2017). *World Population Ageing 2017 - Highlights* (ST/ESA/SER.A/397). Downloaded 3/12/2019 from http://www.un.org/en/development/desa/population/publications/pdf/ageing/WPA2017_Highlights.pdf.

4. "An Aging Nation: The Older Population in the United States," Population Estimates and Projections Current Population Reports By Jennifer M. Ortman, Victoria A. Velkoff, and Howard Hogan. Issued May 2014, downloaded 3/12/2019 from www.census.org.

5. Rane Willerslev, "The optimal sacrifice: A study of voluntary death among the Siberian Chukchi" *Journal of the American Ethnological Society*, November 6, 2009. Downloaded 3/12.2019 from https://doi.org/10.1111/j.1548-1425.2009.01204.x.

6. Sean Rossman. "Americans are spending more than ever on plastic surgery," *USA Today*, April 12,2017, https://www.usatoday.com/story/news/nation...spending...plastic-surgery/100365258/.

7. Chrissy Hayes,"Top 20 Stereotypes of Older People," *The Senior Citizen Times*. November 23, 2011.

8. Ruth A. Lamont "Old Age and Stereotypes" *Psychology Today*, posted February 13, 2015. Downloaded 3/12/2019 from https://www.psychologytoday.com/us/blog/sound-science-sound-policy/201502/old-age-and-stereotypes.

9. Brian Stibich, "How Positive Thinking Can Help You Live Longer" *Verywell Mind*, June 13, 2018. Downloaded 3/12/2019 from https://www.verywellmind.com › Self-Improvement › Brain Health › Healthy Aging.

10. Emmie Martin, "Bankrate: 65% of Americans save little or nothing," CNBC.com https://www.cnbc.com/.../bankrate-65-percent-of-americans-save-little-or-nothing.html. Mar 15, 2018. Downloaded March 14, 2019.

CHAPTER 2: HEALTH MATTERS: FIVE COPING STYLES

1. "Healthy aging into your 80s and beyond," *Consumer Reports*, May 2014. Downloaded 3/12/2019, https://www.consumerreports.org/cro/magazine/2014/06/...your-80s-and.../index.html.

2. "Rate of hearing loss increases significantly after age 90: Hearing aids . . ." https://www.sciencedaily.com/releases/2016/09/160919104555.html.

3. "Healthy aging into your 80s and beyond," *Consumer Reports*, May 2014. Downloaded 3/12/2019, https://www.consumerreports.org/cro/magazine/2014/06/...your-80s-and.../index.html.

CHAPTER 3: UPSIDE DOWN PARENTING

1. Acierno R, Hernandez, M.A., Amstadter A.B., et al. "Prevalence and correlates of emotional, physical, sexual and financial abuse in the

United States: the national elder mistreatment study." *American Journal of Public Health* 100 no. 2, (December 2009): 292–297.

CHAPTER 4: HOLDING ON AND LETTING GO

1. Florida Scott-Maxwell, *The Measure of Our Days* (New York: Penguin Books, 1968). 13ff.
2. William Shakespeare, *King Lear*. Act 5, Scene 3.

CHAPTER 5: FRIENDS

1. Karen Riddell. "Are Our Friends Better for Us Than Our Families?" *Psychology Today*, Posted June 13, 2017. Downloaded March 15, 2019. https://www.psychologytoday.com/us/.../friendship.../201706/are-our -friends-better-u.

CHAPTER 6: LOVE AND SEX

1. Viorst, Judith. *Necessary Losses: The Loves, Illusions, Dependencies, and Impossible Expectations That All of Us Have to Give Up in Order to Grow* (New York: Fireside, 1986) 189.
2. "Intimacy in Later Life," *Easy Living* https://easylivingfl.com/intimacy -later-life/ Feb 10, 2015.
3. Winnie Hu. "Too Old for Sex," *New York Times*, July 13, 2016. A15
4. Emine Saner. "Lust for Life: Why Sex Is Better in Your 80's." *The Guardian*. February 14, 2017.

CHAPTER 7: GRANDPARENTING

1. Robin Marantz Henig, "The Age of Grandparents Is Made of Many Tragedies." *The Atlantic*. Posted June 1, 2018. Downloaded March 15,

2019. https://www.theatlantic.com/family/archive/2018/06/this-is-the
-age-of.../561527/.

2. Paola Scommegna, "More US Children Raised by Grandparents," *PRB*.
March 26, 2012. Downloaded March 15, 2019. https://www.prb.org/us
-children-grandparents/.

3. Emma Elsworth, "Just one in five young people now spend time with
their grandparents," *Independent*, Jan 30, 2018. Downloaded March 15,
2019. https://www.independent.co.uk/.../grandparents-forgotten-young
-people-survey-pensi.

CHAPTER 8: CAREGIVERS

1. "Caregiver Statistics: Demographics," Family Caregiver Alliance,
Downloaded February 26, 2019. https://www.caregiver.org/caregiver
-statistics-demographics.

CHAPTER 9: A SHRINKING WORLD

1. "Aging in Place: Growing Old at Home," National Institute on Aging.
Downloaded February 27, 2019. https://www.nia.nih.gov/health/aging
-place-growing-old-home.

2. "The Village Movement for Seniors," Helpful Village, accessed February
27, 2019. https://www.helpfulvillage.com/the_village_movement.

3. Luke, Helen. *Old Age: Journey Into Simplicity*. Great Barrington, MA:
Lindisfarne Books, 2010.

CHAPTER 10: PAST, FUTURE, AND PRESENT

1. Susan Weinschenk, "The Power of Regret" *Psychology Today*, April 9,
2013. Downloaded February 27, 2019 from https://www.psychologytoday
.com/us/blog/brain-wise/201304/the-power-regret.

CHAPTER 11: DEMENTIA

1. "Dementia Statistics," Clear Thoughts Foundation. Downloaded March 15, 2019 from https://clearthoughtsfoundation.org/living-with-dementia/statistics/.

2. Gina Kolata, U.S. "Dementia Rates Are Dropping even as Population Ages," *New York Times*, November 21, 2016.

CHAPTER 12: TRANSITIONS

1. William Bridges, *Transitions* (Cambridge, MA: Da Capo Press, 2004), 4.
2. William Bridges, *Transitions* (Cambridge, MA: Da Capo Press, 2004), 23.
3. Ashlea Ebeling, "Very Old Folks at Home: Even at 95, Majority Still Live in Homes," *Forbes*, https://www.forbes.com/.../from-homeownership-to-renting-who-is-making-the-switc.

CHAPTER 13: SURVIVOR SKILLS

1. "Income of Today's Older Adults," Pension Rights Center. Downloaded March 15, 2019 from www.pensionrights.org › Get the Facts › Statistics
2. Pindar Quotes (Author of *The Odes*), Goodreads, https://www.goodreads.com/author/quotes/8340.Pindar.
3. Elisabeth Kübler-Ross, David Kessler, et al., *On Grief and Grieving: Finding Meaning of Grief through Five Stages of Loss* (New York: Scribner, 2014).

CHAPTER 14: HOW THEIR KIDS SEE THEM

1. Paula Span. "The New Old Age." *New York Times*, February 20, 2018.
2. Carlson, Elwood. *The Lucky Few.* (New York City, Springer, 2008), 63.

3.   Maria T. Carney, "Elder Orphans Hiding in Plain Sight: A Growing Vulnerable Population," *Current Gerontology and Geriatrics Research.* Volume 2016 (2016), Article ID 4723250.

CHAPTER 15: SPIRITUALITY

1.   Vickor E. Frankl. *Man's Search for Meaning* (New York:Pocket Books 1984).

2.   "The Changing Global Religious Landscape," Pew Research Center. April 5, 2017. Downloaded March 16, 2019 from www.pewforum.org /2017/04/05/the-changing-global-religious-landscape/.

3.   "Connie Goldman's New Book: 'Who Am I . . , Now That I'm Not Who I Was?'" (press release). Downloaded March 5, 2019 from https:// www.prweb.com/releases/2009/10/prweb3004014.html.

CHAPTER 16: APPROACHING DEATH

1.   Moni Basu, "Once taboo, death in America comes out of its shell in unexpected . . ." April 25, 2014. Downloaded from https://www.cnn .com/2014/04/25/living/american-death-customs/index.html.

2.   Olivia Ames Hoblitzelle. *Aging with Wisdom* (Rhinebeck New York; Monkfish Publishing, 2017) 93.

3.   Ann Marie Holland, "The Conversation Project:Sharing Your wishes for the end-of-life" Downloaded March 5, 2019 from https://living.aahs.org /.../the-conversation-project-sharing-your-wishes-for-the-end-of-life.

4.   David Whyte, "Enough," *Where Many Rivers Meet* (Langley, WA. Many Rivers Press, 1998) 2.

CHAPTER 17: UNEXPECTEDLY HAPPY

1. Langer, Ellen J., *Mindfulness*. 25th Anniversary Edition. (Boston: Da Capo Press, 2014) Pgs 82ff.

2. Melissa Dahl, "A Classic Psychology Study on Why Winning the Lottery Won't Make You Happier," January 13, 2016. Downloaded March 15, 2019 from https://www.thecut.com/2016/01/classic-study-on -happiness-and-the-lottery.html.

3. Laura Carstensen: Older people are happier, TED Talk - TED.com, March 13, 2014. Downloaded March 15, 2019 from https://www.ted .com/talks/laura_carstensen_older_people_are_happier?

4. "The Paradox of Aging," Aging Matters. April 25, 2102. Downloaded March 17, 2019 from https://serclab.wordpress.com/2012/04/25/the -paradox-of-aging/.

5. "Emotional Fitness in Aging: Older is Happier," American Psychological Associaton. November 28, 2005. Downloaded on March 17, 2019 from https://www.apa.org/research/action/emotional.

CHAPTER 18: AGING WISELY

1. Erik H. Erikson and Joan M. Erikson, *The Life Cycle Completed, Extended Version* (New York: W. W. Norton & Company, 1997) 61ff.

2. Erik H. Erikson and Joan M. Erikson, *The Life Cycle Completed, Extended Version* (New York: W. W. Norton & Company, 1997).

3. Virginia Woolf, *Mrs Dalloway* (San Diego Harvest HBJ Book, 1925) 79.

CHAPTER 19: THE LUCKY GENERATION

1. Class of '56 Commencement Address, Special Collections Libraries, Smith College, Northampton, MA

2. *TIME* Magazine—U.S. Edition—November 5, 1951 Vol. LVIII No. 19, content.time.com/time/magazine/0,9263,7601511105,00.html.

3. "The Baby Boomer Generation: Baby Boomers Are Reaching Retiring . . ." Seniorliving, Downloaded March 17, 2019 from https://www.seniorliving .org › Life.

4. Elwood Carlson. *The Lucky Few* (New York City, Springer, 2008), 23.

5. Ibid, 132.

6. Ibid, 164.

7. "The Harried Life of the Working Mother," Pew Research Center October 1, 2009. Downloaded March 17, 2019 from www.pewsocialtrends .org/2009/10/01/the-harried-life-of-the-working-mother/.

CHAPTER 20: A NEW VISION FOR OLD AGE

1. "The Polluted Asian City with the Longest Life Expectancy," YouTube https://youtube/c3JRRxxZ3Ig.

2. Becca R. Levy, Martin D. Slade, Stanislav V. Kasl, et al. "Longevity Increased by Positive Self-Perceptions of Aging," *Journal of Personality and Social Psychology*, Vol. 83, No. 2: (2002) 261–270. Downloaded March 15, 2019 from https://www.apa.org/pubs/journals/releases/psp -832261.pdf.

3. Document of responses to Salem's Community Survey sent to author.

4. Selbe Frame. "Julianne Holt-Lunstad Probes Loneliness, Social Connections," *American Psychological Association*, October 19, 2019. Downloaded March 15, 2019 from https://www.apa.org/members /content/holt-lunstad-loneliness-social-connections.

5. John T. Capioppo and William Patrick, *Loneliness: Human Nature and the Need for Social Connection* (New York:W.W. Norton & Co., 2008).

6. Andrew Van Dam. "A record number of folks aged 85 and older are working," *Washington Post*, July 5, 2018. Downloaded March 15, 2019 from https://www.washingtonpost.com/.../2018/.../a-record-number-of -folks-age-85-and-olde...

SUGGESTIONS FOR FURTHER READING

Agrondin, Marc E. *The End of Old Age*. New York: Da Capo, 2018.

Athill, Diana. *Somewhere toward the End*. New York: W. W. Norton, 2009.

Bridges, William. *Transitions: Making Sense of Life's Changes*. New York: Da Capo, 2004

Erikson, Erik H., and Joan M. Erikson. *The Life Cycle Completed*. New York: W. W. Norton, 1998.

Gawande, Atul. *Being Mortal*. New York: Metropolitan Books, 2014.

Gross, Jane. *A Bittersweet Season: Caring for Our Aging Parents and Ourselves*. New York: Vintage Books, 2012.

Gulette, Margaret Morganroth. *Ending Ageism or How Not to Shoot Old People*. New Brunswick, New Jersey: Rutgers University Press, 2017.

Hoblitzelle, Olivia Ames. *Aging with Wisdom*. Rhinebeck, New York: Monkfish Book Publishing, 2017.

Hogan, Paul, and Lori Hogan. *Stages of Senior Care: Your Step-by-Step Guide to Making the Best Decisions*. New York: McGraw-Hill, 2010.

Lake, Helen. *Old Age*. Great Barrington, MA: Lindisfarne Books, 2010.

Langer, Ellen J. *Mindfulness, 25th Anniversary Edition*. Philadelphia: Da Capo Press, 2014.

Lebow, Grace, et al. *Coping with Your Difficult Older Parent: A Guide for Stressed-out Children*. New York: Quill, 2002.

Sarton, May. *Encore: A Journal of the Eightieth Year*. New York: Norton & Company, 1993.

Stahl, Lesley. *Becoming Grandma: The Joys and Science of the New Grandparenting*. New York: Penguin Random House, 2017.

Viorst, Judith. *Necessary Losses: The Loves, Dependencies and Impossible Expectations that All of Us Have to Give up in Order to Grow*. New York: Simon & Schuster, 1986.

Williams, Mark E. *The Art and Science of Aging Well: A Physician's Guide to a Healthy Body, Mind, and Spirit*. The University of North Carolina Press, 2016.

REFERENCES

CHAPTER 1: I AM NOT OLD!

Books

Chittister, Joan. *The Gift of Years: Growing Older Gracefully.* New York: Bluebridge, 2008.

Valliant, George. *Aging Well: Surprising Guideposts to a Happier Life from the Landmark Harvard Study of Adult Development.* Boston: Little, Brown & Company, 2002.

Articles

Depp, Colin, Ipsit V. Vahia, and Dilip Jeste. "Successful Aging: Focus on Cognitive and Emotional Health." *Annual Review of Clinical Psychology*, no. 6 (2010): 527–555.

Graham, Judith. "Getting Rid of the Negative Stereotypes—and Biases—about Aging." *Washington Post*, November 4, 2017. https://www.washingtonpost.com/.../getting-rid-of-the-negative-stereotypes...biases-

Websites

ChangingAging. https://www.changingaging.org.

National Center for Creative Aging. https://www.creativeaging.org.

SeniorPlanet. https://www.seniorplanet.org.

CHAPTER 2: HEALTH MATTERS: FIVE COPING STYLES

Books

Hogan, Paul, and Hogan, Laurie. *Stages of Senior Care: Your Step-by-Step Guide to Making the Best Decisions.* New York: McGraw Hill, 2010.

Morris, Virginia. *How to Care for Aging Parents.* New York: Workman Publishing, 2014.

Articles

Crimmins, Eileen. "Trends in the Health of the Elderly." *Annual Review of Public Health:* no. 6 (2010): 79–98.

Levy, B.R., M.D. Slade, and S.V. Kasl. "Longitudinal Benefit of Positive Self-Perceptions of Aging on Functional Health." *Journals of Gerontology & Psychological Sciences and Social Sciences.* no. 57(2002): 409–17.

Websites

National Council on Healthy Aging. https://www.ncoa.org/healthy-aging.

American Psychological Association, https://www.apa.org/pi/aging/resources/guides.

CHAPTER 3: UPSIDE DOWN PARENTING

Books

Chast, Roz. *Can't We Talk about Something More Pleasant: A Memoir.* New York: Bloomsbury, 2014.

Gross, Jane. *A Bittersweet Season: Caring for Our Aging Parents—and Ourselves.* New York: Random House, 2011.

Articles

Berman, Claire. "What Aging Parents Want from Their Kids." *The Atlantic*, March 4, 2016.

Bookman, Ann and Delia Kimbrel. "Families and Elder Care in the Twenty-First Century." *The Future of Children*. no. 21 (2011): 117–140.

"Wisdom for Adult Children Caring for Aging Parents," *NPR*. January 23, 2012. https://www.npr.org/2012/01/23/.../wisdom-for-adult -children-caring-for-aging-parents.

Websites

AgingCare. https://www.agingcare.com/adult-children-aging-parents.

Adult Children of Aging Parents. https://www.acapcommunity.org.

CHAPTER 4: HOLDING ON AND LETTING GO

Articles

Sheets, Hilarie M. "You Become Better with Age." *Art News*, May 20, 2013.

Shortsleeve, Cassie. "Mindful Aging: What It Is, and Why You Should Be Doing It." *Prevention*. July 28, 2017.

Websites

Next Avenue. https://www.nextavenue.org/what-aging-means-today.

HelpGuide. https://www.helpguide.org/aging.

CHAPTER 5: FRIENDS

Books

Lang, Frieder, and Karen Fingerman. *Growing Together: Personal Relationships across the Lifespan*. Cambridge, UK: Cambridge University Press, 2004.

McFadden, Susan, and John McFadden. *Aging Together: Dementia, Friendship and Flourishing Communities*. Baltimore: Johns Hopkins University Press, 2011.

Articles

Baumeister, R. F., and M. R. Leary, "The Need to Belong: Desire for Interpersonal Attachments as a Fundamental Human Motivation." *Psychological Bulletin*, 117, no. 3 (1995): 497–529.

Neilson, Susie. "In Old Age, Friendships Might Matter Even More Than Family." *Cut*, June 16, 2017. https://www.thecut.com/2017/... /in-old-age-friends-might-matter-even-more-than-family.

Rook, Karen, and Susan Charles, "Close Social Ties and Health in Later Life: Strengths and Vulnerabilities." *American Psychologist*: 72, no. 6 (2017): 567–577.

Websites

Everyday Health. https://www.everydayhealth.com/news/healing-power -friendships-grows-with-age.

CHAPTER 6: LOVE AND SEX
Books

Goldman, Connie. *Late-Life Love: Romance and New Relationships in Later Years*. Minneapolis: Fairview Press, 2006.

Viorst, Judith. *Necessary Losses: The Loves, Illusions, Dependencies, and Impossible Expectations That All of Us Have to Give Up in Order to Grow*. New York: Fireside, 1986.

Articles

Bretschneider J. G., and N. L. McCoy, "Sexual Interest and Behavior in Healthy 80- to 102-Year-olds." *Archives of Sexual Behaviour*: 17, no. 2 (1988): 109–29.

Hu, Winnie. "Too Old for Sex? Not at This Nursing Home." *New York Times,* July 13, 2016, A15.

Websites

Easy Living. https://www.easylivingfl.com.

Senior Journal. https://www.seniorjournal.com.

The Conversation. https://www.theconversation.com/think-youre-not -having-enough-sex-try-being-a-senior-in-assisted-living-72920.

CHAPTER 7: GRANDPARENTING

Books

Isay, Jane. *Unconditional Love: A Guide to Navigating the Joys and Challenges of Being a Grandparent Today*. New York: HarperCollins, 2018.

Articles

Baime, A. J., and Garrett M. Giannella. "Friends for the Ages. The Power of Cross-Generational, Age-Defying Bonds." *AARP The Magazine,* June/July 2017.

Span, Paula. "The Joy of Grandparenting." *The New York Times*, June 7, 2018.

Websites

The Grandparent Effect. Stories from A Quiet Revolution. http://www .grandparenteffect.com/category/news

The Conversation. Why More Grandparents Are Raising Their
    Grandchildren. http://www.theconversation.com/why-more
    -grandparents-are-raising-their-grandchildren-47456.

CHAPTER 8: CAREGIVERS
Books
Hartley, Carolyn, and Peter Wong. *The Caregiver Toolbox*. Maryland:
    Taylor Trade Publishing, 2015.
Hogan, Paul, and Lori Hogan. *Stages of Senior Care: Your Step-by-Step
    Guide to Making the Best Decisions*. New York: McGraw Hill, 2010.
Morris, Virginia. *How to Care for Aging Parents*. New York: Workman
    Publishing Company, 2014

Articles
Kahn, Robin Amos. "The Gift of Caregiving." *HuffPost: The Blog*.
    November 26, 2012. https://www.huffpost.com/entertainment/topic
    /blogs.
Gross, Jane. "An Exercise in Empathy." *The New Old Age Blog, New
    York Times*. Aug. 5, 2008. https://www.nytimes.com/column/the
    -new-old-age.

Websites
Family Caregiver Alliance. https://www.caregiver.org.
Caregiving.Com.https://www.caregiving.com.
AgingCare.Com. https://www.agingcare.com.
ShareTheCare. https://www.sharethecare.org.

CHAPTER 9: A SHRINKING WORLD

Books

Luke, Helen. *Old Age: Journey Into Simplicity*. Great Barrington, MA: Lindisfarne Books, 2010.

Articles

Krystkiewicz, Jill. "Changing Priorities as You Age." *Baltimore Jewish Times*, April 29, 2016.

Luborsky, Mark, Catherine Lysack and Jennifer Van Nuil. "Refashioning One's Place in Time: Stories of Household Downsizing in Later Life." *Journal of Aging Studies*. 25, no. 3 (2011): 243–252.

Websites

Grandparents.com. https://www.grandparents.com/family-and -relationships/caregiving/how-to-downsize.

Time Goes By. https://www.timegoesby.net.

CHAPTER 10: PAST, FUTURE, AND PRESENT

Books

Sawatsky, Jerome. *Dancing with Elephants: Mindfulness Training for Those Living with Dementia, Chronic Illness or an Aging Brain*. Canada: Red Canoe Press, 2017.

Articles

Kotter-Gruhn, Dana and Jacqui Smith, "When Time Is Running Out: Changes in Positive Future Perception and Their Relationships to Changes in Well-Being in Old Age." *Psychology and Aging*, 26, no. 2 (2011): 381–387.

Roese, Neal J., and Amy Summerville. "What We Regret Most . . . And Why," *Personality and Social Psychology Bulletin*, (September 2005): 1273–1275.

Websites

Oprah.com. The Time That Matters Most. https://www.oprah.com /spirit/marianne-williamson-the-time-that-matters-most.

Positive Psychology Program. https://www.positivepsychologyprogram .com/present-moment.

CHAPTER 11: DEMENTIA

Books

Hoblitzelle, Olivia Ames. *Ten Thousand Joys, Ten Thousand Sorrows: A Couple's Journey through Alzheimer's*. New York: Penguin Books, 2010.

Mace, Nancy L. *The 36-Hour Day*, Baltimore: John Hopkins University Press, 2011.

Shouse, Deborah. *Connecting in the Land of Dementia: Creative Activities to Explore Together*. Las Vegas: Central Recovery Press, 2016.

Websites

Dementia Alliance International. https://www.dementiaallianceinternational.org/about-

The MOMA Alzheimer's Project. https://www.moma.org/meetme /index.

CHAPTER 12: TRANSITIONS

Books

Bridges, William. *Transitions: Making Sense of Life's Changes.*
    Cambridge, MA: Da Capo Press, 2004.

Articles

Altman, Rita, "Helping Older Adults Cope with Lifestyle Changes."
    Huffpost: The Blog, December 6, 2013. https://www.huffingtonpost
    .com/entry/lifestyle-change_b_4392546?

Websites

Institute on Aging. https://www.ioaging.org/aging/dealing-unknown
    -transitioning-old-age-gracefully/.

CHAPTER 13: SURVIVOR SKILLS

Books

Kübler-Ross, Elisabeth, David Kessler et al., *On Grief and Grieving:
    Finding Meaning of Grief through Five Stages of Loss,* New York:
    Scribner, 2014.

Articles

"Social Support Activities Lead to Better Quality of Life as One Ages,"
    August 8, 2011.https://www.longtermcarelink.net/article-2011-08-8
    .html.
AgingCare. "Combatting the Epidemic of Loneliness in Seniors," https://
    www.agingcare.com/articles/loneliness-in-the-elderly-151549.html.

Websites

U.S. Census Bureau. https://www.census.gov/.

CHAPTER 14: HOW THEIR KIDS SEE THEM

Books

Berman, Claire. *Caring for Yourself While Caring for Your Aging Parents*. New York: Henry Holt & Company, 2006.

Gastfriend, Judy. *My Parents Keeper: The Guilt, Grief, Guesswork, and Unexpected Gifts of Caregiving*. New Haven: Yale University Press, 2018.

Lebow, Grace and Kane, Barbara. *Coping with Your Difficult Older Parent: A Guide for Stressed Out Children*. New York: Avon Books, 1999.

Articles

Berman, Claire. "What Aging Parents Want from Their Kids." *The Atlantic*, March 4, 2016.

Carney, Maria T. Janice Fujiwara, Brian E. Emmert Jr., et al. "Elder Orphans Hiding in Plain Sight: A Growing Vulnerable Population," *Current Gerontology and Geriatrics Research*, Volume 2016. Article ID 4723250. http://dx.doi.org/10.1155/2016/4723250.

Jefferson, Robin Seaton. "New Survey Finds Adult Children Want Their Parents to Age at Home." *Forbes,* April 30, 2017.

Websites

Adult Children of Aging Parents (ACAP). https://www.acapcommunity.org.

AgingCare. Com. https://www.agingcare.com.

APlaceforMom.com. https://www.aplaceformom.com.

CHAPTER 15: SPIRITUALITY

Books

Reid, Eve. *Fearless Aging: A Journey of Self Discovery, Soul Work, and Empowerment.* North Charleston, SC: Booksurge Publishing, 2007.

Richmond, Lewis. *Aging as a Spiritual Practice: A Contemplative Guide to Growing Older and Wiser.* London: Penguin Group, 2012.

Articles

Park, C. L. "Religious and Spiritual Issues in Health and Aging." *Handbook of Health Psychology and Aging.* New York: Guilford Press, 2007, 227–249.

Laurence, White. "Why Are Old People So Religious?" *Psychology Today*, February 16, 2016.

Websites

Faith, Spirituality and Aging https://www.pbs.org/wgbh/pages/frontline /livingold/etc/faithl.

CHAPTER 16: APPROACHING DEATH

Books

Hoblitzelle, Olivia. *Aging with Wisdom.* New York: Monkfish Book Publishing Company, 2017.

Articles

The American Fear of Death and Dying. *Frazer Consultants.* May 16, 2011. https://www.frazerconsultants.com/fear-death-dying.

Brooks, Arthur C., "To Be Happier Start Thinking about Your Death." Sunday Review. *New York Times*, January 9, 2016.

Websites

Aging with Dignity: Every Life Is Deserving of Dignity. https://www
.agingwithdignity.org.

Five Wishes.https://www.fivewishes.org.

The Conversation Project. www.theconversationproject.org.

CHAPTER 17: UNEXPECTEDLY HAPPY

Books

Carstensen, Laura. *A Long Bright Future: An Action Plan for a Lifetime of Happiness, Health, and Financial Security.* New York: Broadway Books, 2009.

Langer, Ellen J., *Mindfulness, 25th Anniversary Edition.* Boston: Da Capo Press, 2014.

Lustbader, Wendy, MSW. *Life Gets Better: The Unexpected Pleasures of Growing Older.* New York: Penguin Group, 2011.

Articles

Brody, Jane. "Finding Meaning and Happiness in Old Age." *The New York Times* March 19, 2018.

Dahl, Melissa, "A Classic Psychology Study on Why Winning the Lottery Won't Make You Happy," *The Cut.* January 13, 2016. https://www.thecut.com/2016/01/classic-study-on-happiness-and-the-lottery.html.

Fried, Laura. "Making Aging Positive." *The Atlantic.* June 1, 2014.

Szalavitz, Maia. "With Age Comes Happiness." *Time.* Feb. 18, 2013.

Websites

National Council For Aging Care/Aging.com. https://www.aging.com/the-way-of-living-being-happy-and-healthy-at-an-old-age.

Positive Psychology Program.com. https://www.positivepsychologyprogram
.com/positive-aging.

CHAPTER 18: AGING WISELY
Books

Erikson, Erik, and Joan Erikson, *The Life Cycle Completed*. New York:
W. W. Norton 1997.

Hollis, James, Ph.D. *Living an Examined Life: Wisdom for the Second
Half of the Journey*. Boulder, Colorado: Sounds True, Inc., 2018.

Articles

Matthews, Christopher. "Top Ten Books about Growing Old." *The
Guardian*, December 13, 2017.

Leland, John. "The Wisdom of the Aged." *New York Times*, December
25, 2015.

Logan, J. R., R. Ward, and G. Spitze. "As Old as You Feel: Age Identity
in Middle and Later Life." *Sociological Forces* 71 (1992): 451–67.

Websites

The Legacy Project: Lessons for Living from the Wisest Americans.
https://www.legacyproject.human.cornell.edu.

Cornell University Legacy Project Blog. https://www.news.cornell.edu
/stories/2011/08/karl-pillemer-launches-wisdom-website.

CHAPTER 19: THE LUCKY GENERATION
Books

Carlson, Elwood, *The Lucky Few. Between the Greatest Generation and
the Baby Boom*. New York City: Springer, 2008.

CHAPTER 20: A NEW VISION OF OLD AGE

Articles

Van Dam, Andrew. "A Record Number of Folks Age 85 and Older Are Working." *Washington Post,* July 5, 2018.

Websites

AARP Network of Age-Friendly States and Communities Tool Kit
  https://www.aarp.org/livable-communities/network-age-friendly
  -communities/.
World Health Organization, WHO | Towards an Age-Friendly World
https://www.who.int/ageing/age-friendly-world/en/.

Videos

The Polluted Asian City with the Longest Life Expectancy – YouTube, uploaded April 16, https://www.youtube.com/watch?v=c3JRRxxZ3Ig.

ABOUT THE AUTHOR

Katharine Esty is a psychotherapist, a social psychologist, a writer, and a change agent. She has written two previous books, *The Gypsies: Wanderers in Time* and *Twenty-Seven Dollars and a Dream: How Muhammad Yunus Changed the World*. She also co-authored *Workplace Diversity: A Manager's Guide to Solving Problems and Turning Diversity into a Competitive Advantage*. A mother of four sons and a grandmother, and now a widow, she is focused today on creating a new understanding of the possibilities for old age. Esty lives in a retirement community west of Boston.

AUTHOR'S NOTE TO THE PAPERBACK EDITION

Since the first edition of this book appeared in 2019, the pandemic has dramatically changed the lives of eightysomethings. We, like everyone else in this country, have led vastly curtailed lives since March 2020 when lockdowns began. The pandemic continues at a lower level today as I write in May 2022. We older people have been bombarded with dire warnings about how we are most likely to die from COVID-19. And many of us have died. After years of living with the pandemic, some of us feel battered, exhausted, and fearful. I have also observed an amazing resiliency in us. In our long lives, we have necessarily experienced many ups and downs, and all kinds of hardships.

I've also noticed, and research has backed this up, that many of our adult children were more anxious about us getting COVID than we were. After all, we are used to having death as a neighbor. Many of us feel a new hesitancy venturing out into the larger world. But, at the same time, we are more than ready to resume our lives in their fullness. This dichotomy prompted the *New York Times* to ask me to write an opinion piece on the topic. We, elders, are getting a lot of attention, and that's a good thing to my mind because it helps promotes better understanding.

Since the book appeared, I've had some changes in my life. In 2021, I retired from my psychotherapy practice, at age eighty-seven. I play and dance more. I underwent surgery for a blocked intestine and my recovery took several months. Otherwise, I have spent the years happily at my retirement community, sharing my life and my apartment with Peter, my partner of a couple years. I continue to travel, especially when I can see more of my family. I write a monthly blog about aging well that allows me an opportunity to engage with my readers. Thank you if you've responded. I give talks and make media appearances to spread the good news about aging, and overturn the limiting beliefs that diminish elders in our society. I would like to end ageism.

Please stay in touch. You can find my blog on my website, www.katharineesty.com, where you can also sign up for my monthly newsletter or contact me about an appearance.

Follow me on social media:

Facebook: https://www.facebook.com/katharine.esty.79
Twitter: https://twitter.com/esty_phd
Medium: https://medium.com/@katharineesty.com
LinkedIn: https://www.linkedin.com/in/katharine-esty-phd-5161a13a/